Faith and Health:
A Framework
for Christian Nurses

by

Lynda W. Miller
RN, BSN, MSN, Ph.D.

Trafford Publishing
Victoria, BC, Canada

Note for Librarians: a cataloguing record for this
book that includes Dewey Classification and US
Library of Congress numbers is available from
the National Library of Canada. The complete
cataloguing record can be obtained from the
National Library's online database at:
www.nlc-bnc.ca/amicus/index-e.html
ISBN 1-4120-0976-6

Printed in Victoria, BC, Canada

TRAFFORD

**This book was published *on-demand* in
cooperation with Trafford Publishing.**
On-demand publishing is a unique process and
service of making a book available for retail sale
to the public taking advantage of on-demand
manufacturing and Internet marketing. **On-demand
publishing** includes promotions, retail sales,
manufacturing, order fulfilment, accounting and
collecting royalties on behalf of the author.

Suite 6E, 2333 Government St.,
Victoria, B.C. V8T 4P4, CANADA
Phone   250-383-6864
Toll-free   1-888-232-4444
Fax   250-383-6804
E-mail   sales@trafford.com
www.trafford.com/robots/03-1345.html

10   9   8   7   6   5   4   3   2

ABOUT THE AUTHOR

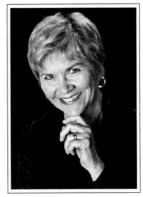

Dr. Lynda W. Miller is a nurse educator and conference speaker who is recognized as a leader in the emerging field of Parish Nursing in both Canada and the USA. In her doctoral research at the University of Victoria, British Columbia, Canada, she developed the first nursing theoretical framework with a clearly Christian faith perspective.

Her publications include articles in *The Canadian Nurse* and *The Journal of Christian Nursing* and a chapter in two edited books: *Promoting Healthy Aging: A Nursing and Community Perspective*, and *Addressing the Spiritual Dimensions in Adult Learning: What Educators Can Do.*

Dr. Miller's professional experience includes hospital, long term care, community health nursing, and independent practice as a wellness educator. She has instructed in four schools of nursing. She has authored and taught courses in Parish Nursing for St.Francis Xavier University (Antigonish, Nova Scotia) Tyndale Seminary (Toronto, Ontario), and Concordia University College of Alberta (Edmonton).

Dr. Miller was a founding member of The Canadian Association for Parish Nursing Ministry and currently serves on their Education Committee.

Her active involvement in the Christian faith community spans fifty years and several church denominations. For the past six years she served in a non-salaried staff position as the Parish Nurse of her local church in B.C. (Brentwood Anglican Chapel).

Born in Pennsylvania, her life has been divided equally between living in the USA and in Canada. She and her husband, Leon LeChasseur, now reside in Victoria, BC (Summer and Fall) and in Solvang, California (Winter and Spring).

Faith and Health: A Framework for Christian Nurses

ACKNOWLEDGEMENTS

To God be the glory. I also want to take this opportunity to gratefully acknowledge the valuable contributions of many people to this book:

First, I give credit to Professor Elaine Gallagher of the Faculty of Nursing, University of Victoria, British Columbia, Canada, who was the academic Supervisor for my doctoral studies. She has been a front-row supporter of me. Without her this book would not have been written.

Two other solid supporters on my dissertation committee were Dr. Harold Coward of the University of Victoria's Centre for Studies in Religion and Society and my external examiner Dr. Ruth Stoll of Messiah College, Grantham, Pennsylvania.

Those who served as critical reviewers of my first draft of the Framework provided crucial feedback for me in the early stage of my research. My faithful prayer partners upheld me through every stage. I've listed all their names in APPENDIX C. Since my graduation Dr. Margaret Myers has urged me on by asking yearly: "Where's the book?"

The artistic talents of Catherine Fraser and Mary Scobie are reflected in my stained glass window figures. The journalistic editing of Suzanne Morphet is evident in CHAPTER 2 and the proficient proof reading of Ann Avery and Linda Ferron is evident throughout the book. The photo on the ABOUT THE AUTHOR page is credited to Mike Mesikep of Los Olivos, California.

Among the people who have exemplified for me what it is to be an "integrator of faith and health" are: Judy Anderson, Ken Bakken, Verna Carson, Jeanne Ensor, Helene Kalsdorf, Phyllis Karns, Marabel Kersey, Judy Shelly, Norma Small, Ann Solari-Twadell, Annette Stixrud and Granger Westberg.

Finally and especially, I want to thank Jeanne Schnell, Eleanor Stamm, Carol Story and my daughter Melody Martin for being so generous with their wisdom and encouragement to me personally over these years.

Faith and Health: A Framework for Christian Nurses

CONTENTS

Faith and Health: A Framework for Christian Nurses

LIST OF STAINED GLASS FIGURES

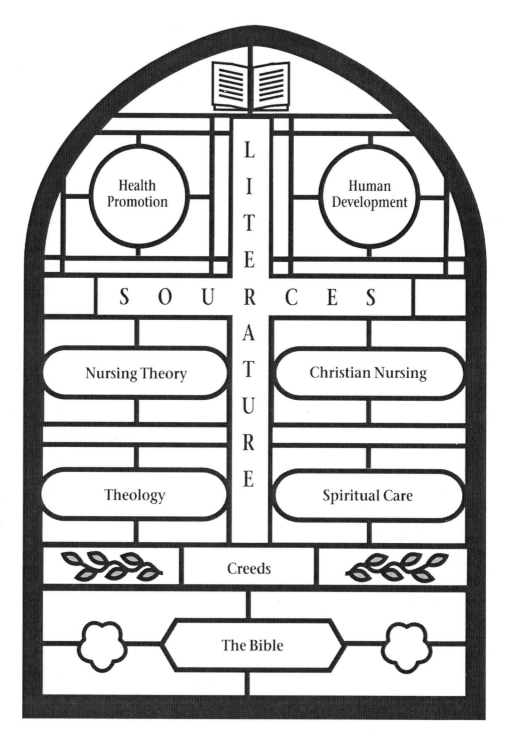

Figure 1: Literature Sources of the Model

Faith and Health: A Framework for Christian Nurses

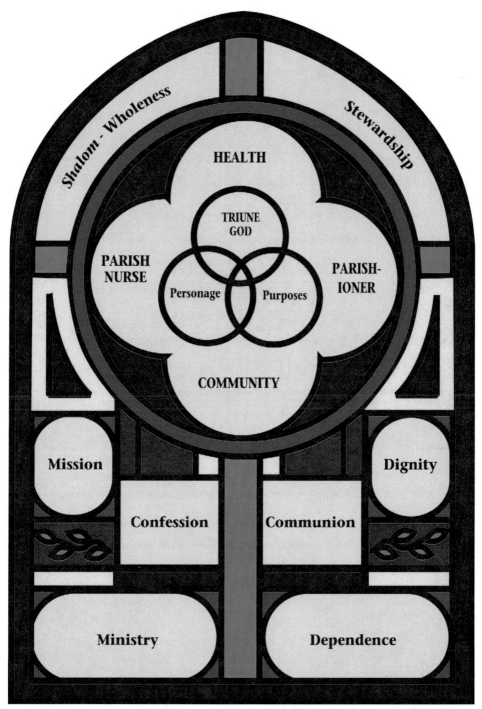

Figure 2: Components and Major Concepts of the Miller Model ©

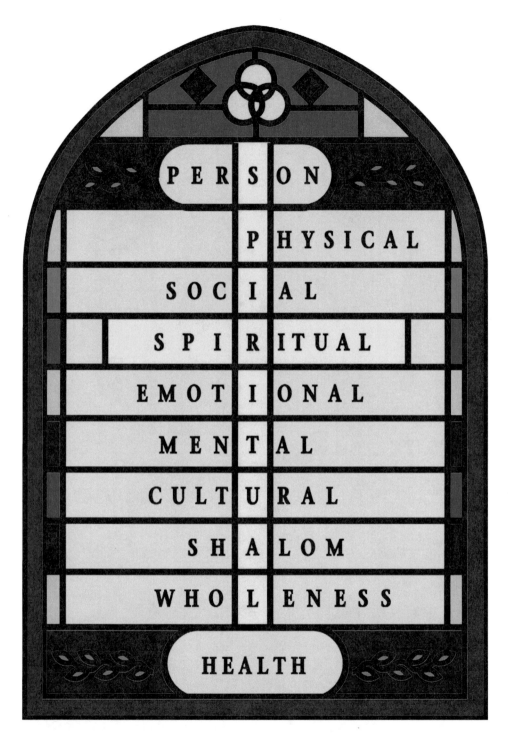

Figure 3: Person and Health – Representation of the spiritual
as integrating all other aspects of the whole person

Faith and Health: A Framework for Christian Nurses

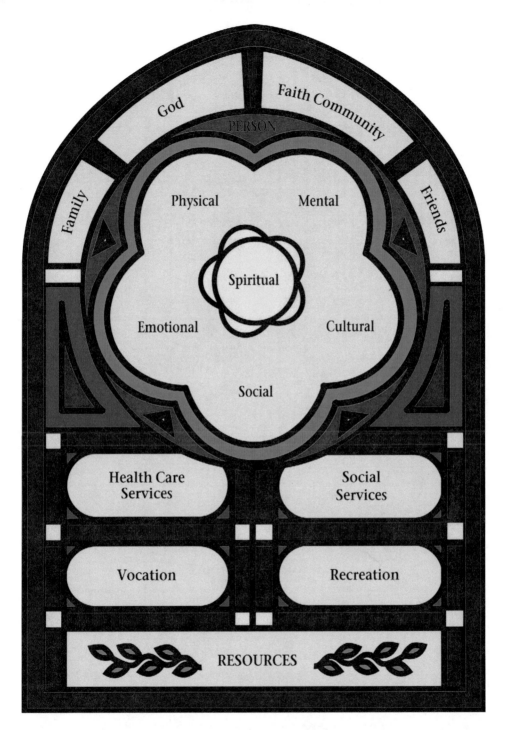

Figure 4: Aspects of the Whole Person
(Spiritual, Physical, Mental, Emotional, Social, Cultural)
and Health Promoting Resources of the Person

Lynda W. Miller

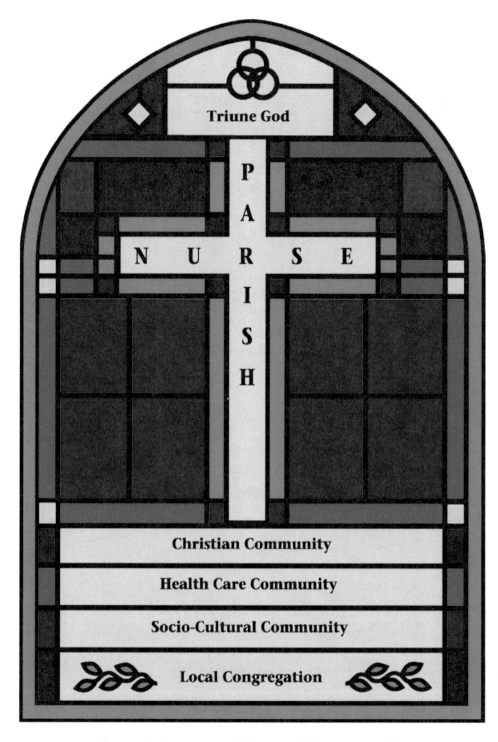

Figure 5: Contexts of the Parish Nurse Role

Faith and Health: A Framework for Christian Nurses

Lynda W. Miller

Faith and Health: A Framework for Christian Nurses

CHAPTER 1: INTRODUCTION

This book is a response to a need. Christian nurses perform their work based on beliefs drawn from their faith, but in the past they've had no specifically Christian theoretical framework to help them. Nurses working in the emerging field of "Parish Nursing" in particular need a framework that helps them explicitly link the concepts of faith and health in their practice, education and research.

I learned of this need when I was introduced to Parish Nursing in 1992. Over the next two years my review of relevant educational materials and publications in the field of Parish Nursing confirmed that need. Since the initial Westberg project in Chicago in 1985 (Westberg, 1990), there has been a rapid expansion of Parish Nursing practice and education, but without enough attention being paid to developing the theoretical base. I found no evidence that existing nursing conceptual frameworks had been critically evaluated as to their relative utility in, or compatibility with, Christian Parish Nursing. No particular existing model had yet become identified with the practice.

Because I was a graduate student in nursing at the University of Victoria at the time, I was able to respond to the need by devoting my doctoral research to intentionally developing a nursing conceptual model from an explicitly Biblical Christian worldview. That dissertation, titled <u>A Nursing Conceptual Model Grounded in Christian Faith</u>, was completed in August 1996. In January of the same year an article I wrote about the model, titled "Nursing Through the Lens of Faith," was published in <u>the Journal of Christian Nursing</u> (Martin, 1996). It was republished in 2002 in an edited book titled <u>Nursing in the Church</u> (Shelly, 2002) (See **BIBLIOGRAPHY**).

Although I had primarily Parish Nurses in mind when I did my research, I believe Christian nurses in a wide variety of practice settings and ministries will also find the Faith and Health Framework a helpful guide for their particular area of practice, education and research. I hope too that the Framework will provide nurses of other faiths a way of identifying the beliefs and values that relate to their own nursing practice.

But the need still continues today, because these publications have not been accessible enough. The bound dissertation is 263 pages long and was written for an academic audience only. A few graduate students have been able to wait long enough to borrow it through the inter-library loan system, but most nursing students and other nurses have had to purchase a copy through me. The journal article provides only a very brief three-page overview of the model. Over the last few years an increasing of number of nurses, in both Canada and the U.S.A., have been asking me: "Do you have a book?" "How can I get it?" That's why I'm publishing it this way now.

So here in this book I describe my original "Miller Model" in depth in an informal "reader-friendly" style. That is what you'll find in **CHAPTER 2**. To depict the Framework in several ways I created, with the help of a commercial artist, five full-color stained glass figures (See **LIST OF FIGURES**). I also wrote a poem as another creative form of expression of the Framework's concepts (See **APPENDIX B**).

Figure 1 depicts the literature sources I surveyed and drew upon in developing the Framework. My primary source was The Holy Bible itself, and thus I have quoted and referenced it extensively. All my quotations are from the New International Version (NIV, 1984), and I've used the NIV's abbreviations for the names of the books of the Old and New Testaments in my citations.

Some relevant textual materials from Christian Church literature, such as creeds, prayers and hymns that I've cited in the book are in **APPENDIX A**. I've also included there an "Historical Background of Parish Nursing" for readers who want to know more about that. Speaking of readers wanting to read more, I provide you with three separate lists. The first one is titled **REFERENCES** and contains all the publications I have specifically cited in the text of this book. The second is titled **BIBLIOGRAPHY**, which are additional readings I haven't cited but I recommend. In **APPENDIX D,** you'll find the third list, which includes various other **RESOURCES**.

CHAPTER 2 will tell you *what is* the "Faith and Health Framework for Christian Nurses." The rest of **CHAPTER 1** will tell you *why* and *how* I developed it. But first, I want to make sure my readers know what these three terms refer to: **worldview, nursing theory,** and **Parish Nursing**.

A **worldview** is a philosophical perspective which includes presuppositions, beliefs and values (Fawcett, 1995; Sire, 1988). More basic and foundational than a conceptual framework, it serves as a frame of reference for all thought and action. An individual's worldview may be more or less conscious, coherent, or consistent (Sire, 1988).

I define **nursing theory** as both *process* and *product*. Both provide a means of viewing phenomena of interest to nursing and of structuring them in useful ways.

My dissertation's definition of **Parish Nursing** is: *a health promotion ministry, based in churches, the focus of which is preventative and in which faith and health are clearly linked and spiritual care is central.* Current definitions of the Canadian Association for Parish Nursing Ministry (CAPNM) are:

> *Parish Nursing* is a health ministry of faith communities which emphasizes the wholeness of body, mind and spirit.
>
> *A Parish Nurse* is a registered nurse with specialized knowledge who is called to ministry and affirmed by a faith community to promote health, healing and wholeness.
>
> The *role of a Parish Nurse* is to promote the integration of faith and health in a variety of ways that reflect the context of the faith community. Specific examples include: health advocacy, health counseling, health education, and resource referral. (See CAPNM under Organizations on the Resources List in **APPENDIX D**).

Parish Nursing in its broadest sense may be practiced in diverse spiritual and religious contexts. For example, the original Christian prototype in the U.S.A. is currently being adopted in some Jewish and Muslim faith community settings. I limited my research, however, to the Christian faith context.

WHY DEVELOP A FAITH AND HEALTH FRAMEWORK?

As I said at the beginning of this chapter, the reason I developed the Faith and Health Framework was because I saw a need. I am aware though that many nurses, including some Parish Nurses, don't think they "need" any nursing theory. It is a common misperception that "the theoretical" is something very separate and different (e.g. done only by "nurse theorists in ivory towers at universities") from "the practical" (e.g. done by "real nurses on the front lines in the real world"). Actually *all* nurses bring theory into their practice, whether or not they are conscious of it, or consistent, or can express it. Theoretical frameworks help nurses make choices, and evaluate, and make changes in their practice. They also provide language for nurses to communicate among themselves and with others what is important to the profession.

In the nursing literature I've reviewed, there is a general consensus that nursing as a profession requires an explicit and sound theoretical foundation, and that it must be continually developed (Fawcett, 1995). For example, both the U.S.A.'s National League for Nursing and the Canadian Nurses Association require as a criterion for accreditation of educational programs a description of their curricula's theoretical framework. The profession's mandate, given by society, is to prepare nurses for roles that are still evolving. This is particularly applicable to educational programs preparing Parish Nurses as theirs is an independent nursing practice.

There are two **underlying premises** to my nursing theory development research work:

1) That nurses' theoretical worldviews affect nurses' professional actions, and

2) That nurses can mutually benefit from the continuing processes of informing and allowing for comparative critiques of one another's conceptual frameworks.

My intention in the dissertation was to "put something on paper" that I hoped would encourage and enhance the thinking, understanding, dialogue, and actions of anyone interested in clearly linking faith and health. My Faith and Health Framework represents a beginning in nursing theory development from a Christian worldview which I hope will encourage further development by others. Why I created it then, and why I'm putting it "out there" in this form now, is because I believe I'm responding not only to a professional need of nurses, but also to a personal spiritual "call" from God to "just do it!"

HOW WAS THE FRAMEWORK DEVELOPED?

The Framework described in **CHAPTER 2** is primarily a product of my own personal process. That process included personal activities of rational inquiry, intuition, meditation on biblical passages, contemplation, and prayer. Another way of describing these activities is to say that both "left-brain" and "right-brain" ways of processing were involved. Academically speaking, my research approach was from the philosophical perspective of the Humanities rather than from the Social Sciences.

My starting point was to raise some research questions for myself to pursue, such as:

- What distinguishes Parish Nursing from other kinds of nursing practice?
- What does the role description of the Parish Nurse as an "integrator of faith and health" involve? (Westberg, 1990, p.37)
- How do I "integrate" my own personal faith and health?
- What does The Holy Bible say about health and wellness?
- What does The Holy Bible say about nursing?

My starting question was the personal one: "How do *I* integrate *my own* personal faith and health?" A dictionary definition of *integrate* (from the Latin *integer* meaning "whole") is *bringing parts together into a whole* (Guralnik, 1975). The development of this model has required the bringing together of a multiplicity and diversity of parts (for example, specific health concepts and faith tenets) from a variety of sources. Because I myself would be one of those sources, my first step was to do some self-reflection and to acknowledge my underlying beliefs and values about:

a) **health promotion nursing**
b) **nursing conceptual frameworks**
c) **Christian faith**

The following is my list of beliefs under each of these three headings:

a) **health promotion nursing**
- The promotion of the health/well-being of individuals, families, and groups is a valued and appropriate Christian nursing practice within faith communities.

- People (e.g., parishioners and Parish Nurses) can be empowered—within their community/church congregation—by health-promoting knowledge, attitudes, actions, and support.
- An independent specialty practice of health promotion nursing (e.g., Parish Nursing) assumes a basic nursing education which meets the licensing requirements and standards of practice for Registered Nurses, plus adequate preparation and experience in family and community health nursing.

b) nursing conceptual frameworks
- Conceptual models reflect worldview attitudes, assumptions, beliefs, and values, which in turn affect actions relevant to health and health care.

c) Christian faith beliefs
- There are some major, basic tenets of the historic Christian faith, relevant to health, about which there is unifying agreement among Christians across cultural and denominational diversity.
- One's conceptions of the Triune God inform all other conceptions of life.
- My life/health is a gift from God with no guarantees and I am entrusted by God with responsibility for the choices I make which affect my life and my health.
- A challenge to my well-being in one area (e.g., spiritual, physical, mental, emotional, social, or cultural) affects, and is affected by, the others in wholly inter-connected ways.
- I live in a loving personal relationship with the Triune God: God(Father)/Christ(Son)/The Holy Spirit as revealed in The Holy Bible and in my own faith experience.
- The Holy Bible is God's Word in written form: inspired, infallible, authoritative and applicable to all areas of life. (For example, my Christian worldview provides moral and ethical guidance in my daily decision making.)
- I also acknowledge here my own bias as a Christian. My personal theological/faith community education and experience (in urban

and suburban churches, ranging in size from 70 to 700 members, in both the U.S.A. and Canada) are primarily from a conservative, evangelical, Protestant perspective.

My research methodology included conducting an extensive search and review of relevant literature. My focus in this review was on identifying concepts of faith and of health, and their interrelationships. For the first three months I studied only The Holy Bible as my primary source. A tool that really helped me was an integrated software program (Biblesoft, 1994) that included several versions, a concordance, a commentary, and dictionaries of Greek, Hebrew, and other biblical terms. I then turned to a wide range of literature sources in nursing theory, human development, theology, health/wellness, and pastoral/spiritual care (See **Figure 1: Literature Sources of the Model**).

Within my review of the nursing theory literature, for example, I looked at the philosophical foundations of the major current nursing models. I also included the work-in-progress of several Christian nurses in the areas of Christian worldview and spiritual care who have published subsequently (See **BIBLIOGRAPHY**). I reviewed materials, dated 1985 to 1995, of various Christian schools of nursing and of Parish Nursing educational and service programs. I reviewed too the printed proceedings of several Westberg Symposia (See International Parish Nurse Resource Center in **APPENDIX D**). In all these materials I identified relevant topics, themes, core curricular concepts, assumptions, values and theoretical materials presented or referenced.

During the four-year period of my graduate studies, I completed the Northwest Parish Nurse Ministries' preparation course through Concordia College in Portland, Oregon, and a theological directed study course in faith, health and aging with Dr. Edwin Hui through Regent College, Vancouver, BC. I attended 10 conferences as a participant-observer. These included one regional and two national conferences on Christian nursing, two regional and five national conferences on Parish Nursing, and one national conference on congregational health ministries. At these events I conducted informal focus groups and interviews with several national leaders in the field of Parish Nursing in the U.S.A. The two key questions I addressed to participants were "What is Christian nursing?" and "How is Parish Nursing distinguished from other kinds of nursing practice?"

Once I'd developed a first draft of the Framework, I circulated it to 24 reviewers, selected for their professional perspectives of either nursing, nursing education, theology, or pastoral ministry. The 17 who provided a critique are listed in **APPENDIX C**). This is what I asked the reviewers to consider and respond to:

      (1) Clarity of concepts

      (2) Internal consistency within the model

      (3) Interrelationships of components and concepts.

      (4) To what extent the model is consistent with your own beliefs, values, assumptions, and Christian worldview.

      (5) Concepts which could be addressed further, or added.

      (6) What you think might be possible implications and useful applications in nursing practice, education, and research.

      (7) What you see as difficulties or limitations.

      (8) Any other comments or suggestions you would like to make.

I made revisions based on their responses, but did not circulate another draft, as I was seeking feedback, not consensus.

During two years of my graduate studies I met on a scheduled basis with an ordained minister/spiritual director for personal spiritual direction, guided meditation and retreat, and for prayer regarding the dissertation work. In addition, throughout the whole time, there were 15 people, mostly nurses, whom I'd drawn from the Christian faith community, who served as my "prayer partners" (See list in **APPENDIX C**). I kept in contact with them regularly, by telephone or in person, individually and occasionally in small gatherings for discussion and prayer. In the final stage of completion of the process, several of them were present and provided prayer support at my oral examination of the dissertation.

Briefly then, in summary, this **CHAPTER 1: INTRODUCTION** has answered the basic questions of *why* and *how* I developed the Faith and Health Framework and has prepared you for **CHAPTER 2's** description of *what* it is. In **CHAPTER 3** we'll consider the question *now what?*

CHAPTER 2: THE FRAMEWORK COMPONENTS AND CONCEPTS

In this book I have included several stained glass window figures designed to represent The Faith and Health Conceptual Framework. In **Figure 2**, you'll see the components of the Framework. Think of these as the center and the outer petals of the flower, keeping in mind that each one is attached to the center and connected to one another. Also like a flower, each component is required for the Framework to be complete. For nurses who have read about other current nursing theories, the labels "person," "health," "nurse" and "community" are familiar, while the terms "parish," "parishioner" and "Parish Nurse" may be unfamiliar even to some Christians. In this chapter, I'll describe each component and discuss its relationship to the others in the Framework.

THE TRIUNE GOD

At the heart of the Faith and Health Framework is **The Trinity:** *God the Father, Christ the Son and the Holy Spirit.* Belief in a Triune God is something that Christians have affirmed through the last twenty centuries. It is absolutely central to the Christian faith. It is what unifies Christians in spite of cultural and denominational diversity. The fact that the God described in The Holy Bible actually exists and that He reveals Himself to people, who are His special creations, are basic tenets taught by all branches of the Christian church. Accordingly, the Trinity is the centerpiece of the stained glass window that is the pictorial representation of the Framework (See **Figure 2: Components and Major Concepts of the Model**).

If you ask me to describe the Trinity, I can't provide a full and complete picture. No person can because our human understanding is finite, and the Trinity is a mystery that hasn't yet been fully revealed. This is pointed out in books from both the Old and New Testament (See Lk. 10:21-22; Eph. 5:32; Job 38:1-4, 42:3b; Ecc. 3:11).

However, using The Holy Bible and two historic creeds of the Christian Church, "The Apostle's Creed" and "The Nicene Creed", one can find the core Biblical truths that distinguish the Christian worldview from all others. Christians around the world still hold these beliefs today. For Christian nurses, these Biblical truths must be known and understood because they are relevant to their everyday work.

These core beliefs focus on who God is and His purpose for us. There is considerable overlap between them because one cannot separate the nature or character of God (His **personage**) from His will (**purpose**).

God's Personage

If you tell someone you believe in God they might very well ask *"What* God do you believe in?" Perceptions of "God" differ greatly among individual members of any given faith community. However, The Holy Bible reveals many aspects and attributes of His nature, more than is possible to summarize here. I venture to say *the Triune God,* as Christians know Him today, *is a personal God who has intimate, loving relationships. He is sovereign, good (in the sense of righteous), just and merciful (or gracious).*

Let's look at the first set of attributes; that the Triune God is a personal God, with intimate, loving relationships. By personal, I mean He is revealed in three persons, as mentioned previously: God the Father, Christ the Son and The Holy Spirit. Imagine three different consciousnesses or one divine consciousness shared by three persons with a "pure reciprocity and perfect harmony both with respect to one another and in their relationships with human beings and the whole of creation" (O'Donnell, 1989, p. 107). In the book of Genesis in the Old Testament, descriptions of the Creation of the world and humankind use the personal pronouns "I" (Ge. 1:29) and "us" (Ge. 1:26) as well as "The Spirit of God" (Ge. 1:2). From a Christian theological perspective, these passages refer to the Trinity.

According to the apostle John, the essential nature of the Triune God is Spirit (Jn. 4:24), but as we know, Jesus Christ was also fully human. In fact, there are frequent references to His "incarnation," a word that is taken from the Latin *caro,* meaning "flesh" (Jn. 1:14; Stein, 1973). The intimate personal relationship God had with the incarnate Jesus Christ is that of Father and Son. Jesus refers to this relationship in His statements that "I and the Father are One" and "...No one comes to the Father except through me" (Jn. 10:30; 14:6, 10-11; Eph. 4:3-6). As a human being Jesus expressed a separate identity in that He frequently prayed to God, including His last prayer, at His death, "Father, into Your hands I commit my spirit" (Lk. 23:46).

This belief in the Trinity is reiterated when Christians read aloud in church from the Apostles' Creed: "I believe in God, the Father Almighty, creator of heaven and earth;" "I believe in Jesus Christ, His only Son, our Lord;" and from the Nicene Creed: "We believe in one God, the Father, the Almighty, maker of heaven and earth, of all that is, seen and unseen. We believe in one Lord, Jesus Christ, the only Son of God, eternally begotten of the Father, God from God, Light from Light, true God from true God, begotten, not made, of one being with the Father (See **APPENDIX A:** Creeds).

The Holy Spirit is also intimately inter-connected with God and Christ. This is apparent in the promises Jesus made to His disciples, both before His death and in appearances to them after His resurrection: "God will give you another Counselor to be with you forever—the Spirit of truth...He lives with you and will be in you. I will not leave you as orphans; I will come to you" (Jn. 14:16-18); "Unless I go away, the Counselor will not come to you; but if I go, I will send him to you...He will not speak on His own...He will bring glory to me by taking from what is mine and making it known to you (Jn. 16:7, 13b-14); "Wait for the gift my Father promised. In a few days you will be baptized with the Holy Spirit (Ac. 1:4-5).

Now let's examine the way in which the Triune God is revealed as sovereign, good, just, and merciful. Throughout The Holy Bible, God is described as the Creator and Sustainer of the universe. This theme is particularly evident in the many references to "The Kingdom of God" (for example, Mt..12:28; Mk. 10:15; Jn. 3:3), which in its essence is the reign, or rule, of God as King in personal relationship with individuals who are His subjects. The picture one sees is of a God who has a loving concern for, and ultimate authority over, all the actions of His universe (Sire, 1988).

The Holy Bible also reveals God's personage as good (or righteous), just and merciful (or gracious) (Dt. 32:4; Ps. 145:9). God is a holy judge concerned with personal and social righteousness. Inherent in these descriptions of the character of God is the existence of a supreme law, His law (Ex. 20). Justice requires a moral foundation and there are moral absolutes of right and wrong within Christianity. The Law of the Old

Testament and Jesus' teachings in the New Testament present specific ethical standards. The Triune God Himself is the standard against which all moral judgments are measured, the fullest embodiment being the person of Jesus Christ (Sire, 1988). Christians know that at Christ's future return He will "judge the living and the dead" (See **APPENDIX A**: The Apostles' Creed; Ac. 17:31a; Jn. 5:27-29).

It is important to note there is no contradiction in the dual beliefs that the Triune God personifies both Love and Judgment. For example, "God hates sin but loves the sinner" is a familiar axiom among Christians. A human analogy is that of parents who demonstrate their love for their children by making their expectations of behavior clear and holding their children accountable (Gaede, 1993).

God's Purpose

With this picture of the character of God, let's look at His will or purpose for us. There are two major beliefs that unify Christians and which are particularly relevant for Christian nurses. These are:

In the Beginning, the Triune God created everything good, intended for harmonious relationships,

and

Since the Fall, restoration of relationships is made possible through Christ's life, death, resurrection, and ultimate return.

Christians today, including Christian nurses and the people they serve, experience tension because they are living, physically and spiritually, in the overlap of these two contrasting worlds. These are described in theological terminology as "the kingdom of light" juxtaposed with "the kingdom of darkness;" that is, world God made juxtaposed with the sin-afflicted world of today, also known as "the kingdom of darkness." (See Jn. 3:19-21; Eph. 5:8-11, 15-16). The "kingdom" viewed as "the reign of God" is in some sense past, present, and future, both now and not yet. We'll discuss implications of this for everyday living later, but first we need to understand God's will as it relates to these two worlds.

According to the Biblical record, the self-existent God brought everything else into being and declared all His creation good (Ge. 1:31; Jn. 1:1-3). Human beings were made "in the image of God" to enjoy harmonious intrapersonal and interpersonal relationships with Him and all of His creation (Genesis 1:27). We were created male and female, in full and equal partnership, with shared responsibility in work and family life, and in stewardship of the natural world (Ge. 1:27-30; 2:18-28; Ecc. 2:24-26, 3:11). God "blessed" human beings (Ge. 1:28).

A publication titled <u>The Christian Humanist Manifesto</u> (Bloesch et al., 1982) talks about God's purpose in creation: "The meaning of human life is moral and spiritual: moral, in the performance of God's will, which is both just and loving; spiritual, in a fellowship with God and other persons...Labor and leisure, science and art, family and state, belong to human life as God meant it to be. Yet the meaning of life is not found in these activities but in the God who enables them" (p. 16).

God created humans to be volitional; capable of exercising the free will He gave us, capable of intellectual and spiritual discernment, and of moral choice. But God did not intend us to be autonomous. Human life is to be received as a gift and responded to in acts of loving worship. Harmonious relationships are to result from continuing dependence on and obedience to the Creator (Ge. 2:7; Ex. 20:2-3; Dt.. 4:39-40; 1 Ki. 3:3,14-15; Ps. 100:3-5; Ro. 1:20).

From the Biblical perspective, moral goodness is seen as human obedience and its consequences. Evil is seen as human (or angelic) rebellion and its consequences (Isa. 14:12-15; Wright, 1992). The disobedience involved in the Fall recorded in Genesis 3 caused damage to all creation, alienation from the Creator, and discord in all relationships (Ex. 34:5-7a; Ro. 3:23, 8:22-23). For example, both the rebellious angelic beings (e.g., Satan) (Rev. 12:9) and humans (e.g., Adam and Eve) presumed to become "like God" and to usurp His authority (Ge. 3:5). Thus, in the present fallen world, the fallen angels and fallen human nature continue to oppose the Rule of God (Jn. 16:8,11b; Ladd, 1974; Rev. 12:17b). The relevance of this theology to the Framework will be discussed later.

Since the Fall, restoration of relationships is made possible through Christ's death, resurrection, and ultimate return. If you think about it, all of the words used to describe God earlier— sovereignty, love, goodness, justice, and mercy—are illustrated by this statement. Both in the Old (First) Covenant between God and His people in Old Testament history and in the

New (Second) Covenant with believers in Christ Jesus, God took the initiative to restore relationships. However, reconciliation requires a personal response of repentance and turning to God in obedience to God's will. This is explained to Christians in what is frequently referred to as "The Gospel of Salvation," which is a translation from the Greek meaning in English "Good News" (Mk. 1:15, 10:15; Mt. 7:21; Jn. 3:3; Ro. 1:16). Though the New Testament's "Gospels" were recorded by these disciples of Christ, Christians believe the Triune God is the author and agent of *The* Gospel.

The simplest description of The Gospel is given by the Apostle John when he wrote: "For God so loved the world that he gave his one and only Son, that whoever believes in him shall not perish but have eternal life" (Jn. 3:16-18). In The Holy Bible, to "believe" is to "take into the heart, to adopt, to feel akin to or morally related to" (Moore, 1993, p. 48). To "believe The Gospel" requires more than intellectual assent to the historical person of Jesus Christ and the historical facts of what He did. The verb "believe" is linked with the Anglo-Saxon words *lief* and *luf*, meaning "to love." The related word "faith" is linked to the Latin *fidere* meaning "to trust" (p. 48). In The Holy Bible, to have faith in Christ is to have a personal relationship that trusts in Him alone for salvation. It involves submission—a surrender of will—to Jesus Christ as Savior and as Lord (Moore, 1993; Wright, 1992).

Another way of summing up The Gospel is to say that for Christians, Jesus is more than a messenger of the gospel; He *is* the gospel" (italics mine) (Lockyer, 1986). The Apostle Paul expressed concern that Christians in the early churches at Colossus and Corinth not be later misled by "deceptive philosophy" or "a different gospel." He wrote to them:

> "I am afraid that just as Eve was deceived by the serpent's cunning, your minds may somehow be led astray from your sincere and pure devotion to Christ. For if someone comes to you and preaches a Jesus other than the Jesus we preached, or if you receive a different spirit from the one you received, or a different gospel from the one you accepted, you put up with it easily enough" (2 Co. 11:3-4)

> "See to it that no one takes you captive through hollow and deceptive philosophy, which depends on human

tradition and the basic principles of this world rather than on Christ" (Col. 2:8).

To conclude, we can state simply: The Gospel is "Good News" because a loving God did for humans what they could not do themselves by providing a way through Christ to restore relationships (Heb. 9:14-15, 22, 26; 1 Jn. 4:10). Having established the center of the Faith and Health Framework in its concepts of the **Personage** and **Purpose** of the Triune God, we are ready to consider the next component of the Framework: **Person / Parishioner.**

PERSON / PARISHIONER

The person component in a nursing conceptual framework is particularly important because the nurse's beliefs about human nature (one's own and others' nature) affect how s/he works with people. How the nurse views human health, aging, illness, suffering, healing, and death impacts nursing care. This Framework also recognizes that people relate wholly to the nurse as co-participants in the process of promoting their health.

Concepts relevant to personhood (of both the nurse and the people with whom the nurse works) are covered in this component, while concepts specific to the working relationship will be discussed later in the component **Nurse / Parish Nurse**

In general, the conceptual frameworks found in the nursing literature define personhood in terms of the individual as an autonomous self. Most reflect a secular humanist worldview in which the human self is central and in which no transcendent sacred "higher power" external to the human self exists. What distinguishes this nursing framework from others is not that it acknowledges a wholistic body-mind-spirit view of person, for various others do as well (Blattner, 1981; Henderson, 1966; Watson, 1988). Many frameworks allow for spiritual care of persons. Most incorporate spirituality within broader psychosocial or culturally sensitive approaches. If you look at nursing education curricula, you will usually find that current conceptual frameworks do two things: They define the spiritual in psychological terms of finding strength, meaning, or hope in the face of illness, suffering, or death, and they treat spiritual care as an "add-on" rather than core content (Miller, 1995; Shelley, 1993).

In this Framework, spirituality is front and center because the Triune God is at its core and because it defines personhood in terms of spiritual relationship with God. It's my premise, the personage and purpose of God, as described in the preceding section, transform people and provide them with more than just a Christian system of thought or philosophical worldview. I rely primarily on Biblical texts that refer to the origin and nature of human beings in relationship. There are two key words to keep in mind in this discussion: they are "dignity "and "dependence".

Dignity

Christians view human beings as specially made "in the image of God" (Ge. 1:27). Human dignities and the related ideas of personal worth, respect, and self-esteem derive from this belief. Dignity also stems from the unconditional love of the Triune God toward all people, and the special covenant relationship with those who accept The Gospel of Christ (Jer. 31:3; Jn. 3:16; Jn. 4:10; Ro. 5:7-8).

From the Creator's perspective, every person (e.g., parishioner and nurse) is valued as a unique, special creation who bears resemblance to Him. That inherent value, regardless of a person's outward appearance or performance, is commonly referred to today as the "sanctity" or "sacredness" of human life and is an acknowledgement of a humanity's inner spiritual nature.

It is important to note that in the Old Testament there is no trichotomy of body, mind, and spirit. In the Genesis account of creation, God first forms the human body from the "dust" (the Hebrew *aphar*) and then blows into the nostrils "living breath" (*ruach*) to animate the body as a "living being" (*nephesh hayyah*) (Ge. 2:7; Isa. 42:5; Robinson, 1946, p. 70). Throughout the Old Testament, the words *ruach* (moving air) and *nephesh* (the organ of breathing) refer to the basic principle and vital power of human life (breath) (Wolff, 1974). *Nephesh* can also be rendered "an inspirited whole" or simply as "person" (Brittain, 1986, p. 107). Biblical scholars tell us these words never referred to an intellectual "mind"—as the Greek word *psyche* represents—or to a disembodied "soul" which exists before birth or after death (Robinson,

1946, p. 70). Scripturally speaking, God created "embodied persons" not spiritual "souls" now captive to physical bodies. Pelikan (1989) further notes that the Genesis 2:7 statement "And man became a living soul" makes clear that man "did not merely possess it, he *became* it (italics mine)...the man in the man" (p. 206).

Biblically defined, every person has a spiritual identity separate from the Creator both before human biological conception and after biological death (Ps. 139:13). The Holy Bible does not fully reveal what life after death is, but the New Testament affirms that individuality continues in new resurrected bodies (Ro. 8:22-23; 1 Co. 15:22-23; 2 Cor. 4:14). Statements from the Christian creeds of this belief are: "I believe...in the resurrection of the body, and the life everlasting;" "We look for the resurrection of the dead, and the life of the world to come" (See **APPENDIX A:** Creeds).

The Faith and Health Framework's concept of the human spirit differs from nursing frameworks whose philosophical base views death either as extinction or as transcendent merging of individual identities with impersonal life force/energy.

Stoll's (1989b) definition states that "man is truly a simultaneously complex, multidimensional person and a unitary organism" whose "differing facets of...personality and life" (as a Christian) are integrated into a whole by "Jesus Christ as Lord and Savior" (p. 162) is consistent with this Framework's definition of human beings as whole persons. Both maintain the central Christian conception of the spiritual dimension as that which animates and integrates all the dimensions of the whole person.

I prefer the term "aspect" to "dimension" because "dimension" suggests quantifiable measurement of separate parts, whereas "aspect" means "a way in which a thing may be viewed" (Stein, 1973). Here, aspect is intended to convey a notion inclusive of the spiritual as well as of the physiological and psychological. In stating the "Greatest Commandment," Jesus uses terms that could be considered four aspects of the person: "Love the Lord your God with all your heart and with all your soul and with all your strength and with all your mind" (Lk. 10:27). Biblically speaking, "heart" refers to the inner being or spiritual nature, while "soul" describes the personality (psychological nature) and "mind" relates to cognition (Mt.

11:29). "Strength" could refer to one's will expressed bodily in physical action.

This Framework contains six aspects (spiritual, physical, mental, emotional, social and cultural) and can be visualized in the accompanying figures.

Figure 3 is a stained glass window with panes in a crossword puzzle configuration. The spiritual is central and connects all other aspects. This figure also represents the inclusion of all six aspects within the Framework's component of health as *shalom*-wholeness, which will be discussed in the next section.

Another way I like to illustrate these aspects is by using the human hand. We can visualize a hand with each of the fingers and thumb representing the physical, mental, emotional, social, and cultural aspects, and the palm of the hand representing the spiritual. Because these may be viewed as parts of a functioning whole, it is a useful metaphor for discussing differing aspects of a person's life or health. For example, as a Parish Nurse, I've found this helpful in assessing parishioners' health-related needs and resources and as a teaching tool. I'm not suggesting that either **Figure 3** or the simple metaphor of the hand adequately represents the complexity of a human being, but both serve to illustrate the major and central place of the spiritual.

In the stained glass window of **Figure 4**, the "rose window" design in the center represents the six aspects of Person/Parishioner and the surrounding panes suggest various types of resources that promote personal health/*shalom*-wholeness. Although the window, like the hand, describes the centrality of the spiritual in integrating all aspects of the person, it too does not adequately reflect interrelationships or the relative contribution of the various resources to promoting health. Just as a hand functions as an interdependent whole, and a stained glass window is composed of interdependent panes, both figures symbolize fully integrated wholeness. This Framework reflects the premise that a challenge to one's personal health in any one aspect affects, and is affected by, every other aspect. Both figures are relevant to all of the Framework's components: **Person / Parishioner, Nurse / Parish Nurse, Health / *Shalom*-Wholeness**, and **Community / Parish**.

Another way this Framework differs from others is in its conception of human beings as "fallen image bearers" (Crabb, 1987, p. 112). This refers to the Christian belief that the human reflection of the divine image of the Triune God has been distorted by the Fall. Every person sins (i.e., "misses the mark" of perfection intended in creation) and no one can earn God's forgiveness or favor, which the just and loving Father offers as a gift through the Son's death and resurrection to those who accept it (Ro. 3:23; 1 Co. 15:21-22; 2 Cor. 5:17; Eph. 2:8-9, 4:22-24; Col. 3:10; I Pe. 1:23). The new biological life of the newborn baby and the renewed spiritual life of the "born-again" believer in Christ are both gifts from the Triune God.

A central theme of <u>The Holy Bible</u> is love, particularly "covenant love." Fallen image bearers are valued primarily because they are loved (Sherburne, 1990; Sire, 1988). The Greek word *agapao* (translated "love" in the New Testament) means to have "esteem or high regard" (Lockyer, 1986). The same word is used to describe both the loving relationship of God the Father toward Jesus the Son and of the Triune God toward people (Jn. 3:16, 14:21, 17:25-26). It is also the basis of the love of Christians for one another (Lewis, 1963; Lockyer, 1986), which we will discuss further in the later component **Community/Parish**.

The Incarnation itself expressed esteem for humanity. In Jesus' life He demonstrated equal regard for all persons and in His death and resurrection equal access to the Kingdom. His gospel message of the Kingdom and His ministry of healing were equally available to all. Jesus' personal relationships—with women, children, and the outcast or despised in Jewish society (e.g., lepers, adulterous women, Samaritans, tax collectors, and Roman soldiers)—were clearly non-discriminatory on the basis of gender, age, ethnicity or social status (Mt. 8:5-7, 12:25; Jn. 4:9-10). He related to people as individuals, as whole persons (body/soul/spirit). He was not only concerned with people's spiritual condition but also addressed their physical health and social and economic condition (Mt. 11:4-5; Wright, 1992). The following passage reflects Jesus' recognition of the plight of fallen image bearers. At the beginning of His ministry, Jesus proclaimed himself as the fulfillment of the following prophecy concerning physical, emotional and social ills:

[Jesus reading from the scroll of the prophet Isaiah:] "The Spirit of the Lord is on me, because he has anointed me to preach good news to the poor. He has sent me to proclaim freedom for the prisoners and recovery of sight for the blind, to release the oppressed, to proclaim the year of the Lord's favor."...[Jesus speaking:] "Today this scripture is fulfilled in your hearing" (Lk. 4:18-19, 21).

An important concept in this component of the Framework is that all persons have intrinsic God-ascribed value and are to be esteemed (by themselves and others) irrespective of their physical, mental, or social status (Taylor, 1986). The expectation that older persons be duly respected and cared for by their immediate family and by members of their faith community is clearly presented in The Holy Bible. One example is the instruction: "Rise in the presence of the aged, show respect for the elderly and revere your God. I am the Lord" (Lev. 19:32). Within "The Ten Commandments" of the Old Testament, the commandment to "honor your father and your mother" is coupled with a promised reward of long life (Ex. 20:12). This injunction to honor one's parents applies not only during childhood but also throughout one's life (Ex. 20:12, 21:17; Lev. 19:3; Dt. 27:16; Pr. 23:22; Mk. 10:19). This injunction is extended in the New Testament to communal caring for all, especially the most vulnerable (widows, orphans, the sick, and the poor) in the church family (Jas. 1:27). The familiar "Golden Rule" (Mt. 7:12) guides Christians to treat all persons as they themselves would like to be treated (Mk. 7:10-13a; I Ti. 5:1).

Dependence

The second major key word or concept of this component is the Judeo-Christian view of persons as being utterly dependent on God. Beyond being the Creator, the Triune God continues to be active in sustaining humans and their world (1 Ki. 3:14; Isa. 46:4; Pelikan, 1989). In the Christian worldview, God is not comparable to a clockmaker no longer involved after starting the ticking. Rather, humans were designed for relationship— personal, cooperative partnership—with their Designer. In this Framework, a core reality of human existence in a fallen world is that there is a deep spiritual hunger for relationship which will only be fully satisfied in heaven (Crabb, 1987). The importance of interdependence in relationships with others will be addressed in the later component Community/Parish. The focus here is on the concept of dependence on the Triune God as Provider. With that in mind, there are two Christian faith beliefs that are particularly relevant to promoting health:

(1) **pardon** and

(2) **presence**.

The following words from a familiar hymn, based on Lamentations 3:22-23, express both of these well.

> "Great is Thy Faithfulness, O God my Father. Thy compassions they fail not. Morning by morning new mercies I see; all I have needed thy hand has provided. Great is thy faithfulness, Lord, unto me! Pardon for sin and a peace that endureth, thy own dear presence to cheer and to guide; strength for today and bright hope for tomorrow, blessings all mine and ten thousand beside! (by T. Chisholm and W. Runyan, 1923, cited in Hustad, 1992, Hymn #60)

(1) **Pardon**. The Parish Nurse conceptualizes the person as a choice-maker: an actor not a mere reactor to the environment. It is important, however, that choices be made in accordance with God's will. Every person has a unique personality and character, which is expressed in that individual's attitudes and actions (Sire, 1988). As fallen image-bearers, humans may arrogantly assert that they are self-sufficient. They may think they have no need for God and may base their behaviors on what feels right or what works for them. This attitude of "I did it my way" is illustrated in The Holy Bible as the foolishness of sheep who, disregarding their shepherd, go their own separate ways (Isa. 53:6; Jer. 2:13).

This waywardness is a sin that grieves God. On one occasion in Jesus' life, He compared His desire to lovingly provide for people (in Jerusalem) to that of a mother hen in spreading her wings over her chicks (Mt.. 23:37). As He recalled the Jewish people's repeated refusals to receive, Jesus wept (Lk. 19:41). If people acknowledge their actions as sin and repent (i.e., turn from going in the wrong direction to following God), God pardons (forgives) them (Ac. 10:43; Ro. 6:14; Heb. 10:1623).

The notion of self-sufficiency is particularly reinforced in North American society by the high value placed on individual autonomy and independence. Closely linked is industrialized society's devaluing view of elderly people as nonproductive and a drain on public resources. People thus may fear unduly the natural aging process and health problems that lead to what society labels a "loss of independence."

The nurse/Parish Nurse's perspective is quite different. The Christian nurse views people as participants in promoting their own health but does not expect them to do it by their own power (physically or psychologically) or on their own (socially or spiritually). The concepts of empowerment and co-participation with others will be discussed later in the component titled **Nurse / Parish Nurse**.

(2) **Presence**. Although a person may be assured of being loved and pardoned by God, there is still the daily reality of living in a fallen world that naturally brings feelings of fear and powerlessness. Christians are to expect difficulty, opposition and suffering as normal experiences in the present age. For Christians in the early Church, suffering and evil did not have to be explained. They were seen as providing practical challenges requiring a response and opportunities for "living in a way more faithful to their new life in Christ" (Hauerwas, 1990, p. 49). In modern society in general and in secular health care science in particular, sickness challenges the cherished presumption that humans can assume control of their existence. Furthermore, suffering such as chronic illness is interpreted as pointless (Becker, 1973). The empirical biomedical model orients practitioners to "delay endings, not to help patients integrate their illnesses and deaths into an ongoing way of life" (Hauerwas, 1990, p. 125).

In Christianity, God is not an "indifferent spectator of human affairs" (Ladd, 1974, p. 332). He has not abandoned the world to self-destruction or evil, and people are not expected to overcome by their own strength (Ps. 34:18, 46:1). Christians are reassured by the knowledge that the power of God is present and actively engaged in the struggle against evil. The forces of evil are submissive to God's ultimate will. Christians can appropriate this knowledge into their daily life struggles and their ministries (Holst, 1982).

The Christian nurse does not present an idealized view of life in this world, but s/he does see human beings as capable of transcending their natural circumstances. Through faith in the sovereignty of God, people can make some sense of the disorder and distress in this world. Awareness of the presence of the Triune God and faith in His power can provide strength, peace and hope in any personal experience. For example, a frail elderly person can draw on spiritual resources to deal with anxieties about being alone and dying. A number of references from The Holy Bible are relevant here. In the Old Testament, Moses declared:

> "Be strong and courageous. Do not be afraid or terrified because of them, for the Lord your God goes with you; he will never leave you nor forsake you....The Lord himself goes before you and will be with you; he will never leave you or forsake you. Do not be afraid; do not be discouraged." (Dt. 31:6, 8)

Psalmists wrote of God as "our refuge and strength, a very present help in trouble" (Ps. 46:1) and of God's promise to "comfort me once again" (Ps. 71:21). Other relevant promises of God are found in the following:

> "Because he loves me, [says the LORD] I will rescue him; I will protect him, for he acknowledges my name. He will call upon me, and I will answer him; I will be with him in trouble, I will deliver him and honor him. With long life will I satisfy him and show him my salvation." (Ps. 91:14-16)

> "Even to your old age and gray hairs, I am he, I am he who will sustain you. I have made you and I will carry you; I will sustain you and I will rescue you" (Isa. 46:4).

Jesus also offered comfort and encouragement in times of trouble. Jesus said:

> "...do not worry about tomorrow, for tomorrow will worry about itself. Each day has enough trouble of its own" (Mt. 6:34).

> "Peace I leave with you; my peace I give you. I do not give to you as the world gives. Do not let your hearts be troubled and do not be afraid" (Jn. 14:27).

> "I have told you these things, so that in me you may have peace. In this world you will have trouble. But take heart! I have overcome the world" (Jn. 16:33).

The Apostle Paul reminds people of the Triune God working in their daily lives when he writes:

> "And we know that in all things God works for the good of those who love him, who have been called according to his purpose.... He who did not spare his own Son, but gave him up for us all—how will he not also, along with him, graciously give us all things?" (Ro. 8:28, 32)

> "...we do not lose heart. Though outwardly we are wasting away yet inwardly we are being renewed day by day" (2 Co. 4:7).

In another significant passage, Paul testifies to the power of prayer in relieving anxiety and providing strength and peace—whatever the circumstances:

> "Do not be anxious about anything, but in everything, by prayer and petition, with thanksgiving, present your requests to God. And the peace of God, which transcends all understanding, will guard your hearts and your minds in Christ Jesus....for I have learned to be content whatever the circumstances....I have learned the secret of being content....I can do everything through him who gives me strength....God will meet all your needs according to his glorious riches in Christ Jesus" (Php. 4:6, 11-13, 19).

In Christian thinking to acknowledge dependence on God is not passive fatalism. The Christian nurse's faith is very different from notions of karma and fate. The latter stresses the inevitability, irrationality and impersonal nature of one's lot in life. Christian faith stresses the reality of an interpersonal love relationship. This kind of dependence is an active turning to God, trusting in God, and a putting into God's hands. The faith and hope that sustain Christians cannot be labeled "blind" because it is evidence-based: it is grounded firmly in the reality of the constancy of God's benevolence (Heb. 1:10-12, 13:8; Demaray, 1975; Miller, 1995). The presence of The Holy Spirit as personal Counselor (in Greek, *parakletos*, "one who speaks in favor of") supports even the act of faith (Jn. 14:16; Stein, 1973). Relevant here is social scientist Maton's (1989) concept of "spiritual support" which he describes as, "[something] perceived in the context of an individual's relationship with God, particularly perceptions and experiences of God's personal love, presence, constancy, guidance, and availability for the self" (p. 319).

To acknowledge dependence on God is also not a denial of personal responsibility. The human response to receiving the benevolence of God is expected to be not only attitudes (e.g., love, gratitude, or worship) but also actions. Some of these actions, particularly as relevant to promoting *shalom*-wholeness (of oneself, others, and the world), are discussed in the next component of the Framework. The next "petal" to mentally picture in a flower representation of my Framework is **Health** or what I call *Shalom-***Wholeness.**

HEALTH AS *SHALOM*-WHOLENESS

Anyone who has reviewed the literature will see that notions of health, wellness, and well-being are exceedingly broad and complex. All three are ill defined and often confused in their application. Originally, the English word "health" meant "wholeness". It derives from an Anglo-Saxon root *hael* meaning "hale" or "whole" (Moberg, 1990, p. 9). The related verb "to heal" connotes "to make whole" (Ott, 1991). Health and healing both originally referred to a fullness of human experience not limited to the physical body. Unfortunately, this is no longer the case. Now society deems people healthy if they are not physically sick. There's another problem with the term health, and that is its application to institutions and medical services that are devoted almost exclusively to treating illness rather than to promoting health (e.g., hospitals being renamed health centers).

"Wellness" is a less problematic term because it is closely identified philosophically with holism (i.e., human body-mind-spirit integration). Christians may be reluctant to adopt the term "wellness" if they negatively associate it with "New Age" philosophy and certain alternative medicine or holistic health therapies. The term "well-being" does not have this negative association and has not been "medicalized." Both "wellness" and "well-being" are inclusive terms that embrace cognitive concepts and concrete activities. "Well-being" is more descriptive of a dynamic process and not as suggestive of an idealized end state.

The term "well-being" is compatible with the earlier described concept of inspirited whole/person (body/soul/spirit) and it reflects the unity and synergy of the physical, mental, emotional, social, cultural and spiritual aspects of life (Tubesing & Tubesing, 1983). Unfortunately, its recent popularity in scientific and lay literature has muddled its meaning. Because of the multiple meanings or lack of distinct definition of the terms health, wellness, and well-being, I've rejected them all and have chosen to define health as **Biblical *shalom*-wholeness** instead.

Before examining what is meant by the Biblical concept *shalom*-wholeness, I think it is important first to address briefly the Framework's view of the relationship between health promotion and healing. The question has been raised whether Parish Nursing's focus on health promotion involves a "rather major shift in the church's tradition" of focusing on healing "as represented by Jesus, the early church, healing shrines, medical missions, and chaplaincy" (T. Droege, personal communication, December 28, 1995). Having reviewed the relevant literature, I'm persuaded that health promotion and healing cannot be sharply distinguished, particularly if what is being "promoted" is understood as Biblical *shalom*-wholeness. To contrast them creates a false dichotomy similar to the expression "cure versus care" which I've often heard applied to the roles of physicians versus nurses. Historically, the church's involvement in promoting health has indeed been less obvious but nonetheless present (K. Bakken, personal communication, January 6, 1996; Bakken, 1992). In recent decades, people's awareness of preventive health measures has increased and that has been reflected by a growing interest among churchgoers in exploring whole-person health within the faith community (Westberg, 1990).

Shalom-Wholeness

The Biblical conception of health is best expressed by the Hebrew word *shalom*, which is translated in English as either "wholeness" or "salvation" depending on the context (Wilson, 1966, p. 19). The Latin word *salvus*, from which the English "salve" and "salvation" are derived, also refers to "wholeness" (Wilson, 1966, p. 19). In the New Testament, the same Greek word is used to mean both "saved" in a theological context and "made whole" or "healed" in a medical context (p. 19). The Biblical conception of sickness (i.e., "dis-ease") is disruption of any dimension of wholeness, and healing is restoration of wholeness (Christian Medical Commission, 1990). In the New Testament the terms "wholeness" and "holiness" are interchangeable (Evans & Small, 1989).

The health component of this Framework is broadly defined as Biblical *shalom*-wholeness. The essence of Biblical *shalom*-wholeness is spiritual and its full meaning, like the conceptualization of the Triune God, is a mystery beyond human comprehension. The closest word to shalom in English, "peace," does not reflect the richness of the Hebrew. *Shalom*'s basic meaning is *dwelling at peace and in harmony in all relationships: within oneself, with God, with other people, and with the created natural world* (Evans & Small, 1989; Tubesing & Tubesing, 1983). This peace comes from loving God and living by His instructions (Isa. 26:3; Lockyer, 1986; Ps. 119:165). The Old Testament meaning was completeness, soundness, and well-being of the total person. In the Old Testament, the word *shalom* is found mainly in prophetic, anticipatory contexts (Isa. 9:67a). In the New Testament, the Hebrew conception of *shalom* is further expanded as the revealing of "The Kingdom of God" through the work of Jesus Christ and of the Holy Spirit (Jn. 14:27, 16:33).

The Holy Bible describes *shalom* in terms of "inner peace" in a personal sense and "peace with justice" in a communal sense (Robinson, 1946, p. 49). Christians are urged to work for the latter; but it is rarely and only temporarily achieved in the fallen world order. Christians frequently attest, however, to a personal *shalom* described as "it is well with my soul," which includes experiences of *faith, trust, forgiveness, joy, and serenity* (Holst, 1982; Lockyer, 1986; Ps. 4:8; Php. 4:6-7, 11-13, 19; Col. 3:15).

The Holy Bible also describes *shalom*-wholeness in the metaphor of Christ as a "vine" and believers as fruit-bearing branches (Jn. 15:4-11). In this image, being whole (well) arises from the vital relationship of the individual branches with the central vine. Jesus described this image in John 15:4-5, declaring:

> "I am the vine; you are the branches. If a man remains in
> me and I in him, he will bear much fruit; apart from me
> you can do nothing."

The healthy growth of the branches is dependent on their vine source and is evidenced by the wholesome fruit produced (i.e., by the Holy Spirit in the lives of the believers) (Christian Medical Commission, 1990). This "fruit of the Spirit" is "love, joy, peace, patience, kindness, goodness, faithfulness, gentleness and self-control" (Gal.5: 22-23). The adjective "wholesome" is not a Biblical term but is applicable here in that its current meaning incorporates both bodily well-being and moral well-being (Stein, 1973).

In other passages *shalom* refers to "completeness" and "perfection" (Bakken & Hofeller, 1988, p. 8). In the Judaic tradition, God valued and desired perfection. For example, the priest who served at the altar, as well as the animal sacrifice itself, were to be without defects (Bakken & Hofeller, 1988; Lev. 21:3; Dt. 15:21). In the New Testament, Jesus Christ's death fulfilled the Law's requirement of the perfect sacrifice (Ro. 8:16; Heb. 9:11, 10:18; Gal. 3:10-13; 1 Ti. 3:16) and established the new and better covenant which made it possible to be "made perfect" (Heb. 10:14) through Him (Heb. 7:25, 8:6; Ro. 8:16; Php. 1:6, 3:12). The Greek term *teleios* used in these passages and in Jesus' exhortation to "be perfect as your heavenly Father is perfect" (Mt. 5:48; 2 Pe. 3:14-15a) does not mean perfection as purity but translates to "bring to completion" (Bakken, 1992, p. 8). The process of bringing to completion is life-long, involving growth through self-discipline and through the guidance of the indwelling Holy Spirit. It is a process of maturing, of being "imitators of Christ" (2 Cor. 3:17-18) and "growing up in His likeness" (Eph. 4:13)

In this Christian Framework, the idea of well-being as Biblical *shalom*-wholeness is necessarily Christ-centered and faith-centered. As discussed in the previous sections on the **personage** and **purposes** of the **Triune God,** the original plan was that human beings and all of creation would enjoy full and harmonious life (i.e., well-being). The Genesis description of Adam and Eve living harmoniously, walking and talking with their Creator in a world, which was deemed "very good" (Ge. 1:31), could be considered a Biblical Framework of well-being (Ott, 1991). The Fall brought disorder, disharmony and death. Through Christ, personal *shalom*-wholeness became possible, though it cannot be fully experienced in the fallen state of life on earth (Ro. 5:1-2; Col. 1:16-22). By Biblical definition, personal *shalom*-wholeness is possible only through personal relationship with Christ. The ultimate well-being of the human community (full completion of God's shalom) will come only as part of the peace and harmony of all creation after Christ's return. This future "new heaven and new earth" is referred to in Revelation 21:1 (Bakken, 1992; Lockyer, 1986; Rev. 21:1-5a; Ro. 8:20-23; 2 3:13-15a).

On the part of individuals, the personal faith needed to achieve *shalom*-wholeness must be active and willful "confidence" or "trust" (from the Latin *fiducia*) not mere intellectual "belief" (from the Latin *assentio*) (Robinson, 1946, p. 105). It presupposes acknowledgement of one's **dependence** on the Triune God to satisfy the deepest longing in what The Holy Bible refers to as one's "innermost being" (from the Greek *koilia*, literally meaning open space or cavity; metaphorically, a void or empty space to be filled) (Crabb, 1987, p. 105; Jn. 7:37b-38). Such faith makes it possible to be "fully alive": that is, to live life with "enthusiasm," a word derived from the Greek *en* and *theos* (Stein, 1973) meaning a state of being "in God," "full of God" and "in God's fullness" (Eph. 3:19, 4:13). This Christian concept of *shalom*-wholeness as fulfillment is also reflected in Jesus' own statement of purpose: "I am come that they may have life, and have it to the full" (Jn. 10:10).

Valuing of the human body is inherent in the above discussion on the inspirited whole/person. Jesus himself responded to the physical needs of people for food and for healing (Brittain, 1986; Mt. 14:14-16, 11:4-5). The importance of caring for one's body is also iterated in the following two Biblical passages:

> "After all, no one ever hated his own body, but he feeds and cares for it, just as Christ does the church—for we are members of his body " (Eph. 5:29-30).

> "Do you not know that your body is a temple of the Holy Spirit, who is in you, whom you have received from God? You are not your own; you were bought at a price. Therefore honor God with your body" (1 Co. 6:19-20).

From a Christian perspective the health of the physical human body is valued but never viewed as an end in itself or as an object of ultimate concern. As one Biblical scholar has stated, the body is viewed as an "agency for the projects of the total self, to provide a fit instrument for the growth and maturation of men and women in community with others and communion with God" (A. C. Outler, cited in Ott, 1991, p. 49). A Christian's body is never to become an idol. Indeed, one's health may even need to be sacrificed for the sake of a higher good (Bouma, Diekema, Langerak, Rottman, & Verhey, 1989; I Ti. 4:7-8; Heb. 13:16; Ro. 5:7; Mt. 10:37-39; Jn. 12:25). A relevant quotation here is:

> "Therefore I urge you, brothers, in view of God's mercy, to offer your bodies as living sacrifices, holy and pleasing to God—this is your spiritual act of worship. Do not conform any longer to the pattern of this world, but be transformed by the renewing of your mind" (Ro. 12:1-2a).

A Christian's personal faith experience and personal health experience (i.e. *shalom*-wholeness) cannot be separated. This truth is reflected by writers of the New Testament who used words meaning health, wholeness, healing, salvation and holiness interchangeably. The Judaic tradition strongly related bodily health to moral health (Job 7:20; Ps. 38:3, 41:13, 73:3, 16-18, 107:17; Isa. 38:16-17). In the New Testament, references to the human experiences of sickness and death continue to be closely associated with sin. When people asked Jesus specific questions on the subject His responses challenged the early Hebrew belief that personal sin, or God's punishment of it, is always the cause of sickness and death (Lk. 13:4; Jn. 9:2-3). As discussed earlier, sin—whether a specific sin of a person, the sin of humanity in general, or the evil forces at work in the world—impacts the well-being of people today, as it did in Jesus' time, and will until the end of time (Rev. 21:4). No one as a fallen image-bearer living in a fallen world can yet experience perfection or be unaffected by struggles and suffering of some kind (Gal. 5:16-17; Ro. 8:1-6; 2 Co. 12:9-10).

Faced with human frailty, the Triune God is always gracious. Jesus demonstrated this in His response to the disciples who failed to keep watch with Him and fell asleep: "The spirit is willing but the body is weak" (Mt. 26:38, 41). Regardless of the cause of suffering, however, Christians are accountable (as stewards) to promote health/*shalom*-wholeness in themselves, in others and in their community as best they can (1 Co. 6:19-20;

2 Cor. 4:5, 7; Eph. 5:29-30; 1 Th. 5:23; 1 Pe. 2:9-10). With the struggle may come the personal experience of the paradox of Christian living described by the Apostle Paul as "when I am weak, then I am strong" (2 Co. 12:7b-10). For Paul, living the Christian life in his human body was to have a "treasure" (i.e., knowledge of Christ) in a "jar of clay" (2 Co. 4:7). There is also an acknowledgement of human dependence on the Triune God as the source of health/*shalom*-wholeness in Paul's benediction:

> "May God himself, the God of peace, sanctify you through and through. May your whole spirit, soul and body be kept blameless at the coming of our Lord Jesus Christ" (1 Th. 5:23).

Stewardship

Shalom-wholeness also involves the challenge of the balancing act of caring for oneself while caring for others. This is an ongoing concern throughout a Christian's life and is inherent in the concept of **stewardship**. Although the term "stewardship" (from the Greek *oikonomia)* appears infrequently in The Holy Bible, the concept is clearly expressed in both the Old and New Testaments (Christopher, 1990). Human stewardship is to be a reflection of the Triune God's own compassionate concern for the well-being of all Creation. The "dominion" and "rule" over the created world that God gave to humans, as recorded in Genesis (Ge. 1:26-30, 2:15), was intended to sustain the created world benevolently as He does (Green, 1994). To be a "steward" means to be entrusted with something valuable and to be accountable for it (Lockyer, 1986). Old Testament principles of stewardship include caring for the land, preventing poverty, using God-given skills in His service, and balancing work and rest (Christopher, 1990; Ex. 20:9-10; Ps. 116:16; Pr. 3:5-8).

Examples of stewardship in the New Testament include showing compassion for the poor, demonstrating forgiveness in relationships, being accountable and managing wisely whatever one has received from God (Christopher, 1990; 1 Co. 4:1-2; I Ti. 4:7-8; Heb. 13:16; Jas. 3:17; 1 Pe. 4:10-11a). The Christian view of all of nature as being created by God and belonging, with humankind, to God's kingdom, implies specific obligations for Christians to live in ways which use—but do not in any way abuse—their natural environment (Coward, 1993). Thus, loving concern for promoting health of people encompasses environmental health.

The above principles apply generally both to people as individuals and as members of communities. The concept of stewardship in the latter context will be addressed further in the discussion of Community/Parish and will be applied more specifically to nursing in the Nurse/Parish Nurse section.

Before one can fully understand stewardship as it relates to health/*shalom*-wholeness in this Framework, it's critical to understand the idea of discipline as instruction. The term discipline commonly carries an incorrect negative connotation of punishment, but by dictionary definition, discipline is "to bring to a state of order and obedience by training and control" (Stein, 1973). The word "discipline" derives from the Latin *disciplina* meaning instruction and is equivalent to the Latin *discipul(us)* meaning disciple (Stein, 1973). In The Holy Bible the term "disciple" is rare in the Old Testament (the Hebrew *immud*, rendered "one instructed," in Isaiah 8:16) (Unger, 1961, p. 265). However, the term is common in the New Testament, particularly in reference to the followers of Jesus (the Greek *mathetes*, rendered "learner" and meaning "one who professes to have learned certain principles from another and maintains them on that other's authority," for example in Matthew 5:1-2) (Unger, 1961, p. 265).

Christians are called to **live a life of love** (Eph. 5:2a). This is a disciplined life of seeking to "find out what pleases the Lord" (Eph. 5:10; Heb. 13:16) and not "grieving the Holy Spirit" (Eph. 4:30). For Christians the guiding principle is to be "imitators of God" (Eph. 5:1). Humans loving one another imitate the loving relationship within the Triune God (Jn. 17:24-26). Jesus provided His disciples a human role model of *shalom*-wholeness in living a life of love. When asked which of God's laws was the most important, His reply was:

> "Love the Lord your God with all your heart and with all your soul and with all your mind. This is the first and greatest commandment. And the second is like it: Love your neighbor as yourself" (Mt. 22:36-38).

Jesus clearly linked obeying God's law of love with the experience of joy:

> "As the Father has loved me, so have I loved you. Now remain in my love. If you obey my commands, you will remain in my love, just as I have obeyed my Father's commands and remain in his love. I have told you this so that my joy may be in you and that your joy may be complete. My command is this: Love each other as I have loved you*" (Jn. 15:9-12).

Jesus even declared love to be that which would distinguish Christians:

> "A new command I give you: Love one another. As I have loved you, so you must love one another. By this all men will know that you are my disciples, if you love one another" (Jn. 13:34-35).

The importance for Christians to live a life characterized by love is reiterated in the following quotations from Luke, Paul and John:

> [Jesus speaking] "Which of these three do you think was a neighbor to the man who fell into the hands of robbers?" The expert in the law replied, "The one who had mercy on him. " Jesus told him, "Go and do likewise" (Lk. 10:36-37).

> "The entire law is summed up in a single command: Love your neighbor as yourself" (Gal. 5:14).

> "...and now these three remain: faith, hope and love. But the greatest of these is love "(1 Co. 13:13).
> "If anyone has material possessions and sees his brother in need but has no pity on him, how can the love of God be in him? Dear children, let us not love with words or tongue but with actions and in truth....This is the command: to believe in the name of his Son, Jesus Christ, and to love one another as he commanded us" (I Jn. 3:17-18,23).

> "We love because he first loved us....And he has given us this command: Whoever loves God must also love his brother" (1 Jn. 4:19, 21).

The first step to one's living a disciplined life of love is being restored in a personal loving relationship with the Triune God. This step is followed by the life-long, day-by-day experience described in the New Testament as "keeping in step with the Spirit" (Gal. 5:25) (See also Gal. 5:16-17; Col. 3:12-14; 1 Ti. 4:7-8; 3 Jn. 1:2). This is the same relationship mentioned earlier when we talked about the Triune God being a personal God in intimate, loving relationship.

One of the ways we show appreciation for God's loving relationship with us is through **stewardship** (worship and showing gratitude are examples of other ways). In turn, the desire of Christians (i.e., disciples) to demonstrate love in faithful stewardship of their own bodies and of the human and material resources that have been entrusted to them, strongly motivates them to stay healthy.

Throughout history, The Holy Bible has guided Christians in their efforts to achieve health. Hygienic practices which aid in disease prevention, such as the washing of hands and clothing and the burial of excrement, are described in Lev. 15:8 and Dt. 23:12-13. Also included are prohibitions regarding both under and over eating, the consumption of certain meats, and the overindulgence in intoxicating drinks (Lev. 11:6-8; Pr. 23:20-21; Ecc. 2:24-26, 3:12-13, 8:15). A final example is the balancing of work and rest through the Sabbath Day (one day of rest from work in every seven days) and the Sabbatical Year (one year of rest for cultivated land every seven years) (Ex. 20:9-10; Ecc. 3:12-13, 5:12; Lev. 25:4-5, 23-24; Dawn, 1989).

There are specific commandments against human attitudes and behaviors (i.e., sin) which are contrary to the nature of the Triune God and which cause personal sickness and social disharmony: for example, commandments against adultery, lying, and stealing (Ex. 20:14-16; Eph. 4:25-31, 5:3-5). There are also instructions for practices that promote harmony (i.e., well-being) in relationships, such as showing kindness and forgiveness:

> "Therefore, as God's chosen people, holy and dearly
> loved, clothe yourselves with compassion, kindness,
> humility, gentleness and patience. Bear with each other
> and forgive whatever grievances you may have against
> one another. Forgive as the Lord forgave you. And over
> all these virtues put on love, which binds them all
> together in perfect unity." ...And whatever you do,

whether in word or deed, do it all in the name of the Lord Jesus....(Col. 3:12-14, 17a).

"Do not let any unwholesome talk come out of your mouths, but only what is helpful for building others up according to their needs, that it may benefit those who listen....Be kind and compassionate to one another, forgiving each other, just as in Christ God forgave you" (Eph. 4:29, 32).

There are a number of the classical spiritual disciplines which the church historically has encouraged Christians to use to promote their health/*shalom*-wholeness, including worship (personal and congregational), solitude, meditation, prayer (alone and with others), confession, guidance (e.g., through a "spiritual director"), fasting, study of <u>The Holy Bible</u> (alone and with others), celebration of the sacraments, the practice of "laying on of hands", social fellowship, the practice of "sharing the peace" (i.e., exchange of the traditional greeting "the peace of the Lord be with you" and/or the kiss of peace), hospitality, tithes and offerings, submission to those in authority, living in simplicity, and serving (Bakken, 1992; Whitney, 1991; Wilson, 1966).

NURSE / PARISH NURSE

As a nurse who views nursing through the eyes of Christian faith I have been asked: "Is there a difference between Christian / Parish Nursing and other nursing?" My answer is "Yes, most definitely, but the two are not always distinctly different." This section talks about why that is and about the concepts that differentiate Parish Nursing from secular nursing.

Definitions of the term "Parish Nursing" are provided in **CHAPTER 1**. For the convenience of readers I've repeated them here. My own original **definition of "Parish Nursing"** is:

> "*a health promotion ministry, based in Christian churches, the focus of which is preventative, and in which faith and health are clearly linked and spiritual care is central.*"

Additional definitions I later helped develop for the Canadian Association for Parish Nursing Ministry (CAPNM) are:

> *"Parish Nursing is a health ministry of faith communities which emphasizes the wholeness of body, mind and spirit. Rooted in the vision of Christ as Healer, this ministry grows out of the belief that all faith communities are places of health and healing and have a role in promoting wholeness through the integration of faith and health."*

> *"A Parish Nurse is a registered nurse with specialized knowledge, who is called to ministry and affirmed by a faith community to promote, health, healing and wholeness."*

As clear as these definitions sound, I acknowledge it's often difficult to separate specific concepts that are distinctively Christian from those which characterize current secular nursing in North America in general. This is partly because the historical roots of nursing as a profession today are so tightly intertwined with nursing as a Christian vocation (Shelly, 1994; Taylor, 1986). The difficulty of separating concepts in respect to spiritual care, for example, points to some common ground shared by all nurses sensitive to the spiritual dimension of humans and of health, regardless of their individual worldviews (Carson, 1993). Certainly, Christian nurses do not have the "corner" on caring. However, as this Framework is built on a foundation of which Christ is the "cornerstone" (Eph. 2:20), the concepts of the Nurse/Parish Nurse component reflect the strong ethic of caring inherent in the Christian worldview.

The Christian faith is both philosophical and practical, as is Parish Nursing. In the human person, there is no separation of spirit/soul/body. In daily Christian living, there is also no separation of the sacred from the secular, in that all human work—such as nursing work—is endowed by the Triune God with spiritual significance; the transcendent resides in the common and ordinary aspects of life (Demaray, 1975). The person who is a Christian (by profession of faith in Christ) and is a nurse (by professional licensure in society) expresses the philosophical in the practical.

All of the concepts of human personhood—already discussed in the sections on the **Triune God**, **Person/Parishioner** and **Health/***Shalom-*

Wholeness—are applicable to the nurse/Parish Nurse as a person. That is, every Christian nurse is a whole person and fallen image bearer who is a co-participant (with the Triune God, other individuals and groups) in promoting health (Biblical *shalom*-wholeness and stewardship) of self, of other persons, and of the wider community in which that nurse serves.

Now let's focus on how all of these concepts specifically relate to the role, functions, and key characteristics of Parish Nursing practice. In discussing their work, Christians, including Parish Nurses, often use the words **mission** and **ministry**. We'll use these same terms, the first to address the philosophical *why* and undergirding motivation of Christian nursing in general, and the second to address the pragmatic *what* and *how* of Parish Nursing practice.

Mission

When Christians talk about their "mission in life," they're often talking about their vocation, their calling or their motivation to service. The term "mission" is derived from the Latin *mittere* meaning "to send out," particularly to perform a special duty (Lockyer, 1986). The related term "vocation" (from the Latin *vocare*, "to call") in a Christian context means a calling from God to a holy purpose to which one's life is devoted (Lockyer, 1986). Florence Nightingale, recognized as the founder of modern nursing, recorded her own calling in a diary entry on February 7, 1837: "God spoke to me and called me into His service" (cited in Collins, 1985, p. 5). (See also **APPENDIX A**: "Florence Nightingale Pledge" and "A Quotation of Florence Nightingale")

Examples of mission as calling of people to fulfill specific purposes of the Triune God are found throughout both the Old and New Testaments. These include prophets and leaders of the nation of Israel, Jesus' disciples and other members of the early church (Isa. 6:8; Est. 4:14; Jn. 15:15-16, 21:16; Ac. 2:36, 16:10; Ro. 1:1). The concept of calling can be applied to all Christians in the general sense that the Triune God has a claim on the life of every person who receives salvation. Jesus himself fulfilled a mission—"to seek and to save" (Lk. 19:10) and "to serve" (Mt.20: 25)—which He instructed His disciples to continue. Jesus declared:

"As the Father has sent me, I am sending you" (Jn. 20:21).

"I tell you the truth, anyone who has faith in me will do what I have been doing. He will do even greater things than these" (Jn. 14:12).

"You are the salt of the earth.... You are the light of the world. A city on a hill cannot be hidden. Neither do people light a lamp and put it under a bowl. Instead they put it on its stand, and it gives light to everyone in the house. In the same way, let your light shine before men, that they may see your good deeds and praise your Father in heaven" (Mt. 5:13-16).

The Parish Nurse is sent out both by God and by the congregation. Anglican clergyman Alistair Petrie observes that "people whom God appoints, He also anoints with the spiritual gifts necessary for the task to which they are appointed" (personal communication, November 1995). Particular spiritual gifts of a Parish Nurse might include teaching, healing, giving generously and encouraging (Ro. 12:611b, 13). I'll talk more about the role of the Parish Nurse in the section on **Ministry**.

Even Christians who don't receive a particular calling from God have a meaning and purpose in life. Because the human body is "the temple of the Holy Spirit" (1 Co. 6:19-20), the Triune God is present in all of a Christian's being and doing. Thus, personal endeavors are given meaning by transcendent goals, and every act of Christian service, no matter how small, has significance as activity of the Kingdom of God in the present age (Harakas, 1990; Miller, 1995). Jesus' teaching on this concept altered traditional Jewish understanding by equating service to God with service to others (Lockyer, 1986). **Caring** was given new meaning and consequence when Jesus declared:

"I was hungry and you gave me something to eat, I was thirsty and you gave me something to drink, I was a stranger and you invited me in, I needed clothes and you clothed me, I was sick and you looked after me, I was in prison and you came to visit me.... I tell you the truth, whatever you did for one of the least of these brothers of mine, you did for me" (Mt. 25:35-36,40).

"If anyone gives even a cup of cold water to one of these little ones because he is my disciple, I tell you the truth, he will certainly not lose his reward" (Mt. 10:42).

The work in India of Mother Theresa, who has been quoted as saying, "the poor are our Lord" (Tower, 1987, p. 199), is an example of service rendered to others as to Christ himself. This conception is commonly applied by Christian nurses to their nursing work. One Parish Nursing educational program even describes its theoretical base as "The Mother Theresa Framework" (A. Stixrud, personal communication, June 1994).

A point for Christian nurses to note is that The Holy Bible instructs believers to continually examine their motivation to service. As fallen image bearers struggling with negative forces within and without, their motives may not be pure. Good works are viewed in the New Testament as integral to living out the Christian faith. They are also not onerous obligations and are not to be done to earn favor either with God or other people (Green, 1994; Mt.. 6:1-4). Rather, they are practical expressions of love and gratitude in response to and in reflection of the character and purposes of the Triune God.

Viewed as a calling, Parish Nursing arises from more than mere sense of duty or from awareness of human need. It means more than simply doing the job (Shelly, 1994). In contrast, if caregiving is motivated by the Parish Nurse's own need to be needed or to be controlling of the attitudes or behaviors of other people, it is self-gratifying and selfish: it becomes self-serving. The example of Christ's caring is self-less serving.

True service, Biblically speaking, is done "to the glory of God alone" (in Latin, *soli gloria Dei*) (1 Cor. 10:31; 1 Pe. 4:11). The apostle Paul makes this clear in saying: "whatever you eat or drink or whatever you do, do it all to the glory of God" (1 Co. 10:31), and in urging Christians to "live a life worthy of the calling you have received...[and] be completely humble and gentle; be patient, bearing with one another in love" (Eph. 4:1-2). The connection between acts of giving to others and the experience of having received from God is clearly expressed in the statement: "We love because he [God] first loved us" (1 Jn. 4:19) and in Paul's declarations:

"For we are God's workmanship, created in Christ Jesus to do good works, which God prepared in advance for us to do " (Eph. 2:8-10).

"Each one should use whatever gift he has received to serve others, faithfully administering God's grace in its various forms. If anyone speaks, he should do it as one speaking the very words of God. If anyone serves, he should do it with the strength God provides, so that in all things God may be praised through Jesus Christ" (1 Pe. 4:10-11a).

Within the faith community itself, Christians are often called to specific roles and functions. This leads us to **Ministry**: the *what* and *how* of Parish Nursing.

Ministry

In The Holy Bible, the terms "minister" and "servant" are interchangeable and are applied to a variety of official and lay roles. The use of the word "ministry" today in its broadest sense denotes both "the service to which the whole people of God is called, whether as individuals, as a local community, or as the universal Church," and "the particular institutional forms which this service may take" (World Council of Churches, 1982, p. 21). It includes proclamation of the gospel in both word and works of service. There are differences of opinion among theologians along denominational lines regarding whether clergy and laity should all share in all forms of ministry (e.g., liturgical and pastoral functions) (Shelly, 1995c). There are some churches today that still do not permit women to hold certain positions of authority. I have not yet found in the literature an analysis of how these respective views of ministry may affect the role of the Parish Nurse.

The concept of ministry is expressed very clearly in the New Testament description of a *doulos*, translated from the Greek as "a bondslave". In Biblical times, this was a slave who was offered freedom but who voluntarily surrendered that freedom in order to remain a servant (Lockyer, 1986; Mt. 20:26). Instruction given to members of the early church who were literally slaves or servants also applied figuratively to all members.   In writing to the church in Ephesus, the apostle Paul advises slaves to:

> "Obey your earthly masters with respect and fear, and with sincerity of heart, just as you would obey Christ. Obey them not only to win their favor when their eye is on you, but like slaves of Christ, doing the will of God from your heart. Serve wholeheartedly, as if you were serving the Lord, not men, because you know that the Lord will reward everyone for whatever good he does, whether he is slave or free " (Eph. 6:5-8).

Jesus taught His disciples to serve in the same manner in which He himself was a servant fulfilling His purpose in the Kingdom of God. He countered the typical way human beings "lord it over" those under them (Mt. 20:25) with the challenge "not so with you" (Mt. 20:26) and offered an alternative. Jesus said:

> "Instead, whoever wants to become great among you must be your servant, and whoever wants to be first must be your slave—just as the Son of Man did not come to be served, but to serve, and to give his life as a ransom for many" (Mt. 20:26-28).

> "I no longer call you servants, because a servant does not know his master's business. Instead, I have called you friends, for everything that I learned from my Father I have made known to you" (Jn. 15:15-16).

Jesus both redefined servanthood and showed how to put it into practice within His own intimate loving relationship with the Triune God. Later the apostle Paul reminded all believers their own attitudes should be "the same as that of Christ Jesus: Who, being in very nature God, did not consider equality with God something to be grasped, but made himself nothing, taking the very nature of a servant" (Php. 2:5-7). (See also **APPENDIX A**: "Servant Song".)

Jesus modeled a radically different way of being with people than the accepted norm of society then (and today). He related to each person with the respect shown between equals, the concerned interest between neighbors, and the love between friends. It is this model of mutually serving one another that Christ directed His disciples to emulate (Fordyce, 1990; Green, 1994; Mk. 10:43-45; Lk. 10:36-37; Jn. 13:14-15; Ro. 12:6-11; Php. 2:5-7;).

However, in applying the concept to Christian nursing today, a couple of problems arise.

First, the term **servanthood** carries negative connotations. Given the human history of oppression—especially of women, including at times within Christianity itself—the idea of servanthood is not a popular notion. It is highly unpopular, in fact, in present-day North American society in general and in the nursing profession in particular. North American culture today generally values individualism so highly it is accepting of motivations that may be self-gratifying and assertiveness that may be self-centered. In such a cultural climate, the Biblical concept of self-sacrificing ministry may be difficult for Christian nurses to defend in their practice settings (Miller, 1995). The concept of self-sacrificing ministry in this Framework, however, suggests neither a demeaning role of submissive servitude nor surrender of the nurse's voice (Haugk, 1984).

The second problem arising from the concept of servanthood as it applies to Parish Nursing is that the reality is far from the ideal. Current estimates are that only half of practicing Parish Nurses are being paid. Is Parish Nursing then another unpaid or underpaid (relative to the public or private sector) role for women? Certainly there is heightened sensitivity today to implied power differentials associated in the labeling of particular roles as "women's work." As approximately 98% of Parish Nurses are women, the over-riding concern that women not be exploited to do free work must be addressed in evaluating paid versus unpaid positions. The Holy Bible speaks to this point in supporting workers as deserving of pay for their services to others. For example, the Mosaic Law states in Deuteronomy 25:4 "Do not muzzle an ox while it is treading out the grain." In the New Testament, both Jesus and Paul quote this commandment and apply it to people. In Lk. 10:7, Jesus declares, "the worker deserves his wages." Paul, in letters to early church congregations, asks the rhetorical question, "Is it about oxen that God is concerned?" and immediately answers "Surely He says this for us" (1 Co. 9:9-14). Paul then makes application to both the work of plowmen and threshers and to the work of church elders (1 Ti. 5:17-18) and others (including women, such as Phoebe) (Ro. 16:1-2) who served in teaching and preaching the gospel. He argues strongly that Christians who minister within the church have "the right of support" and should "receive their living from the gospel," just as the Hebrew temple servers "share in what is offered on the altar" (1 Co. 9:9-14). If parish health ministry would be true to this Biblical valuing of all workers and to Jesus' inclusive way of being and working with (ministering to) people, then Parish Nurses would be appropriately valued and adequately paid.

A further point could be made that doing nursing work from altruistic motives and being paid are not incompatible concepts in the church community. As I've said before, within the Christian worldview there is no separation of secular work from sacred work.

For this Framework, a different term than "servanthood" is needed. Defining Parish Nursing work as **ministry** is certainly compatible with beliefs and practices of the present day Christian faith community. I will discuss nursing in relation to that context in the final component of the Framework.

Now that we've defined what ministry is in general, let's look at what roles and functions ministry can take in the church. There is much in the New Testament regarding specific ministries in the early church. These are still relevant to the nurse/Parish Nurse today, both as individuals in the church family and as professionals in their official leadership positions. In the book of Ephesians, Paul lists a number of roles and functions along with their associated spiritual gifts:

> "It was He [Christ] who gave some to be apostles, some to be prophets, some to be evangelists, and some to be pastors and teachers, to prepare God's people for works of service, so that the body of Christ may be built up until we all reach unity in the faith and in the knowledge of the Son of God and become mature, attaining to the whole measure of the fullness of Christ....From Him the whole body, joined and held together by every supporting ligament, grows and builds itself up in love, as each part does its work" (Eph. 4:11-13,16).

> "There are different kinds of gifts, but the same Spirit. There are different kinds of service, but the same Lord. There are different kinds of working, but the same God works all of them in all men. Now to each one the manifestation of the Spirit is given for the common good. To one there is given through the Spirit the message of wisdom, to another the message of knowledge by means

of the same Spirit, to another faith by the same Spirit, to another gifts of healing by that one Spirit, to another miraculous powers, to another prophecy, to another distinguishing between spirits, to another speaking in different kinds of tongues, and to still another the interpretation of tongues. All these are the work of one and the same Spirit, and he gives them to each one, just as he determines" (1 Co. 12:4-11).

"We have different gifts, according to the grace given us. If a man's gift is prophesying, let him use it in proportion to his faith. If it is serving, let him serve; if it is teaching, let him teach; if it is encouraging, let him encourage; if it is contributing to the needs of others, let him give generously; if it is leadership, let him govern diligently; if it is showing mercy, let him do it cheerfully. Love must be sincere...serving the Lord....Share with God's people who are in need. Practice hospitality" (Ro. 12:6-11b, 13).

The role of the Parish Nurse in its broadest sense is as an "integrator of faith and health" (Westberg, 1990, p. 37). It is this central focus and the related emphasis on spiritual care that distinguish Parish Nursing from other types of health promoting nursing practice, such as occupational health or community health nursing. Defining health in the Biblical terms of *shalom*-wholeness also distinguishes the goal of Parish Nursing practice.

As an integrator of faith and health, the Parish Nurse must work closely with the parish pastor. This requires compatibility and effectiveness on the nurse's part, along with a clear sense of the mission and goals of the parish as a whole. Both must also understand their respective leadership roles and be able to address such delicate issues as accountability, confidentiality and the overlapping of roles (Belleau & Warskow, 1995). Roles in a parish, as elsewhere, are defined both by education and by expectation. Although full cooperation, not competition, is intended, tensions may arise if members of the congregation or the parish staff have different expectations or perspectives than the shared ministry team (Djupe, 1990).

The specific roles of each Parish Nurse typically involve health education, counselling, advocacy and linking people to resources, but will vary from nurse to nurse depending on the congregation and community within which she's working.

Parish Nursing is frequently described as a specialized independent practice. In none of the roles and functions is the nurse autonomous. There is shared responsibility and accountability among clergy, lay leaders and church members (Bakken, 1992; Shelly, 1994). There is also close collaboration with others in diverse health-related roles in the wider community. Viewed from the spiritual perspective, the Parish Nurse also acts with, and is ultimately accountable to, God. Stated in the terminology of this Framework, the Parish Nurse is **called** to **stewardship** in one particular **ministry** among the many ministries expressing the work of the Kingdom in the world today.

Professional **competence** is inherent in this Framework's concept of ministry. To adequately fill Parish Nursing roles and functions is a challenge that requires a solid foundation of relevant nursing knowledge and skills consistent with current professional standards of practice. At present, Parish Nursing educators recommend preparation at the baccalaureate level and a minimum of five years experience, plus the completion of an introductory course specific to Parish Nursing (Solari-Twadell, McDermott, Ryan, & Djupe, 1994; Health Ministries Association, 1998; Canadian Association for Parish Nursing Ministry, 2004). A good working knowledge of The Holy Bible and comfortable familiarity with the particular faith beliefs, traditions and practices of the congregation are important. It is also essential that the Parish Nurse's life evidence moral character and a personal faith relationship with Jesus Christ (Shelly & Miller, 1991).

Concepts Central To Parish Nursing

All of the concepts we've talked about earlier apply to Parish Nurses either as individuals or as professionals working with people. But after reviewing the literature on the subject and conferring with practicing Parish Nurses, I've identified the following four concepts as central to Parish Nursing viewed as Christian ministry:

1. (1) **love,**
2. (2) **gracious compassion,**
3. (3) **co-participation,** and
4. (4) **spiritual care.**

(1) **Love**. Love is the bedrock of the Christian faith and central to Christian nursing. The Parish Nurse reflects the character and purposes of God when love is the inner motivation and outer expression of the practice. We talked earlier about Christians as fallen image bearers and the kind of love God has for them. This is Biblical agapao love experienced in intimate relationship with the Triune God and fellow members of the Christian faith community. It is not superficial sentimentality or simply "being nice to the old people." It is seeing in every person what the Triune God sees: a dignity that comes from being loved by the Creator and the Savior. It is acknowledging the realities of people's lives as imperfect, fallen image bearers, struggling in a fallen world. It is also demonstrating gracious compassion.

(2) **Gracious Compassion**. The Christian nurse who acts from the above conception of love can reflect something of the gracious compassion of the Triune God (2 Co. 1:34). The word "compassion" derives from the Latin *com + pati* meaning "to suffer with" and is closely related to compatibility, meaning "going well together with" (Lockyer, 1986; Stein, 1973). Synonyms include "mercy" and "tenderness." Gracious compassion encompasses attitudes and actions: of the head, the heart, the hands and the spirit. It implies a strong desire to alleviate the suffering itself and/or to remove the causes (for example, by advocacy and social activism) (Donley, 1991). It has been described as "compassionate accompaniment" (Donley, 1991, p. 179). This requires of the nurse a capacity both to feel with and be with people. Gracious compassion transcends human empathy because the Holy Spirit is actively involved.

Compassion defined in this way is costly. It requires a willingness by the Parish Nurse to feel something of the vulnerability, loss, or alienation parishioners feel during and after experiences that affect their health/*shalom-*

wholeness. Since the nurse enters into the process as a whole person, the nurse takes the risk of being wounded. Gracious compassion also implies a willingness to make some sacrifice, to go beyond expected norms. It stretches helping as part of the job to "going the second mile" (Mt. 5:41) (Green, 1994; Thomasma, 1994).

(3) **Co-Participation**. Nursing in North American society today is considered a helping profession and the helping relationship is regarded as integral to nursing itself (Adam, 1991; Travelbee, 1966). In this Framework, the concept of helping implies that the Parish Nurse will co-participate in promoting Biblical *shalom*-wholeness and stewardship in self, in other individuals, in families, and in the wider community in which she serves. As noted earlier, co-participation in this context also involves the Triune God.

How effective the Parish Nurse is depends largely on the quality of the helping relationship the nurse has with the person or people in need. Clearly, s/he is only as helpful as the individual or family or group perceive the nurse to be. The cautions raised earlier regarding nursing from one's own "agenda" are relevant here.

Professional competencies are obviously important too, particularly the nurse's skills in communication. Included in this is communication with the Triune God. Praying for oneself, praying for and with others, and teaching people to pray are all essential to care that is spiritual (Gustafson, 1993; Peterson, 1994).

Key to co-participation in a working relationship is the focus on shared process. That is why in this Framework, the term "parishioner" is used to refer to all persons (individuals, families, and groups) with whom the Parish Nurse works, rather than the terms "patient" or "client". I do not use the term "patient" because it is associated with a relatively powerless and passive role as a recipient of care within a medical care delivery system. Although "client" does not have the same associations as "patient," it also does not connote a relationship of equals. Relating to others as parishioners helps the Parish Nurse avoid these pitfalls because she is perceived as "one of us." Because the Parish Nurse's role is based within local congregations and the Christian faith community, the sense of "we-ness" is enhanced, furthering the co-participation process.

The following quote is taken from an interview (E. Gallagher, personal communication, 1992) with an older person who is reflecting on her experience at a Seniors' Wellness Center. I'm including it here because it illustrates well the concept of co-participation in this Framework:

> "I didn't feel anybody was preaching at me at all—I felt like [the nurse] was one friend telling another—which is marvelous when you think of it! PROFESSIONALS, if you please, talking to ME, not like to a bar of soap! At eye level—which is the only comfortable place to live. I learned that here. It makes sense—good sense—common sense. No, I don't think it's common at all—I rarely find it! [laugh]"

This quote also shows how co-participation is **empowering**. Viewing a person as an active co-participant, rather than as a passive patient, discourages a tendency for the nurse to be ascribed a higher status or authority as the perceived health expert who "has the answers" and should "know what's best" for others. The Parish Nurse can be professionally competent at an expert level (as described by Benner & Wrubel, 1984) yet not be the expert in the helping relationship. In this Framework, all of the co-participants are experts and teachers of one another. The relationship is not viewed in terms of the roles of "helper" and "helpee" and certainly not as "fixer/fixee" or "healer/healee."

Empowerment is a key concept in the current literature of gerontology and health promotion (Labonte, 1989). Generally, it is defined in terms of the secular humanist worldview. Empowerment within the Christian worldview, on the other hand, reflects the earlier discussed relationship of human beings as dignified, dependent, image-bearers with the omnipotent Triune God.

There are important differences between this particularly Christian understanding of empowerment in relation to health and the general secular notion. A Parish Nurse helps parishioners identify their needs, goals, strengths, resources and options, and also helps them acquire the necessary attitudes, knowledge, tools, skills and support. This applies equally to a nurse's function in a secular setting. The secular nursing Frameworks view the self—alone or in conjunction with others—as responsible for personal empowerment. They also value maximizing one's sense of personal control.

By contrast, Christians view personal control to the exclusion of the sense of God's control (i.e., His benevolent will) as a negative attribute (Maton & Rappaport, 1984). The metaphor of independently "pulling up one's own bootstraps" is inconsistent with the Christian tenet of dependently drawing closer to the Triune God as the only source of truly transforming power. In Parish Nursing, it is also recognized that health-related experiences that empower parishioners in the direction of living more Christ-like lives are more important than the experience of health *per se*.

Inherent in Parish Nursing practice is recognition of the Parish Nurse's and parishioner's mutual **dignity** and mutual **dependence** as finite fellow beings in loving relationship with the infinite Triune God.

The mutual bond of fellowship (in Greek, *koinonia*) within a congregation, a concept that will be discussed further in the next component of The Framework, is also empowering.

(4) **Spiritual Care**. In this Framework, who the Parish Nurse is as a whole person (spirit/soul/body) is more salient than what the Parish Nurse does in the professional role. Traditionally a nurse's focus has been on tasks. This is clearly reflected in the job lists included in Parish Nursing program design and evaluation reports in the literature. In this Framework, *being* is stressed more than *doing*. A familiar maxim that could apply here is: "Who you are speaks so loudly I can't hear what you're saying." Stated positively in theological terms, the Parish Nurse promotes *shalom*-wholeness of parishioners by living out the Gospel in partnership with God. In practice, the nurse may be caring (being) by not caring (not doing): that is, by sitting still and being still, thus creating sacred space for the Holy Spirit's ministry.

My review of nursing literature concluded that relatively little attention has been given in nursing to the spiritual dimension. There is also little consensus in the nursing literature about the concepts of spirituality and spiritual care (Emblen, 1992). In one sense, all interactions between Christian nurses and the people with whom they are working are spiritual because the human spirit of each person and the Holy Spirit are present. The nurse's caring can also be deemed spiritual when it is demonstrating in some way the character and purposes of the Triune God.

More specifically, spiritual care refers to actions that address an individual's spiritual beliefs, values, and faith practices. This includes finding spiritual meaning in life events which impact health. It also includes identifying and using various spiritual resources to promote, maintain or restore health. These resources include, but are not limited to, (a) personal inner resources (such as spiritual gifts); (b) other people; (c) devotional and worship materials and activities (e.g., Sacraments); and (d) the Triune God. Spiritual care thus is applicable to every person, including the nurse.

The nursing concept of **spiritual care** in this Framework is closely linked to the ministry of pastoral care, which is particularly identified with the roles of the Christian clergy (specifically pastors, ministers, priests and missionaries), as well as with chaplains, pastoral counselors and spiritual directors. Like other leaders in the church, a Parish Nurse must be qualified to offer spiritual care. An intention to provide opportunities for nurses to increase their knowledge and skills in this area is reflected in the recently published guidelines for Parish Nursing educational programs. They recommend curriculum components comparable to clinical pastoral education programs for chaplains (SolariTwadell et al., 1994).

Spiritual care is a shared ministry with those in other pastoral roles and with all who are co-participants within the Christian community/parish. It is central to Parish Nursing. This is evident in the following comments made by an older parishioner about his Parish Nurse:

> "Without the Parish Nurse Program some of us would be poorer in body and spirit. But with it there comes a feeling that God is near—that He comes and loves, that He heals and redeems. My wife and I have had various illnesses that seem to come with the aging process. We have been under the care of our Parish Nurse ever since this program was begun five years ago. We look forward to her visits, because she comes on behalf of the Church, not only with medical knowledge and skill, but also with compassion and love which are uplifting and sustaining" (Nelson, 1990, p. 287).

COMMUNITY / PARISH

A nurse's parish or community might at first appear to be limited to the immediate church congregation. However, this Framework considers not just the physical location of the church and parishioners but the whole environment in which the Parish Nurse is practicing health promotion. All the contexts are viewed from the nurse's perspective. In other words, whatever is labeled "parish" is determined by the parameters of the Parish Nurse role. The parish may mean the local church congregation and its church-related activities. Or, it may mean the larger parish with which the local church is identified denominationally and/or ecumenically. Parish in this sense is generally defined in terms of geographical regions or organizational structures. On another level, the Church worldwide is a further Christian context. There is, in addition, the immediate context of the socio-cultural community. This community context includes cultural norms, and public and private sector resources relevant to Parish Nursing. (See **Figure 5: Contexts of the Parish Nurse Role**) In this section, key concepts relevant to **Community / Parish** are discussed.

In The Holy Bible, "church" and "congregation" are translations of the Greek *eklesia*. "Ecclesiology" refers to studies related to the church (Lockyer, 1986). A present-day description of the Christian Church that I find relevant is: "an international, multiracial community of forgiven sinners [which]...despite failures, inconsistencies, and hypocrisies has pioneered a many-sided humanitarianism" (Bloesch et al., 1982, p. 18). The local church is the visible operation of the Church in a given time and place (Lockyer, 1986). Brueggemann's (1976) concept of "*shalom* community caring" (p. 182) is included in his description of **Christian community** as:

> "a network of persons in covenant with each other, who have made solemn promises to one another about sustaining and caring, defending and enhancing one another. Community is enhanced when all its members are seriously committed to the well-being of all. Conversely, community is diminished when some members hold out on others, set themselves above others, or just plain don't care" (p. 181).

Also relevant is Anderson's (1990) definition of a faith community because it reflects both individual and societal contexts: "An assembly of people whose beliefs about God combine with a common identity, a shared history, regular worship and common values, in order to effect personal and social transformation" (p. 264).

The term "parish," derived from the Greek *paroikos* meaning "neighbor," refers today to the inhabitants and activities of an ecclesiastical district (Stein, 1973). In Christian usage, "parishioner" may also be translated "sojourner," reflecting the view of one's physical life on earth as a temporary stay in one place within the eternal spiritual Kingdom.

Whatever the terminology, promoting health and healing are integral to the Church's **mission** and **ministry**. When local church congregations reflect Jesus' example and teachings, they are by definition "communities of health and healing" (Droege, 1995, p. 117). Churches are concerned about the health of their members and the health of the communities in which they are located (Droege, 1995; Evans, 1995). As stable and respected institutions in society representing all social strata, they provide social as well as spiritual resources for individuals and families across all ages and life stages. Congregations promote health both in philosophical ways (e.g., nurturing spiritual values) and in practical ways (e.g., sponsoring health-related programs) that can have an impact on the health of people and their environment.

Regarding the natural environment, the following basic tenets foundational to the Christian worldview have already been discussed in previous sections:

- *In the Beginning, everything in the natural world was created by the Triune God and declared "good."*
- *The Creator entrusted humans to be guardians and caretakers of the natural environment.*
- *Since the Fall, all of creation suffers negative consequences (e.g., abuse and destruction of land, vegetation, and animals).*
- *All of creation will be restored in the future when the "Kingdom of God" is ultimately established.*

The term "environment" is also used in health-related literature to refer to the physical surroundings in which people live. These include the essentials that support human life (e.g. air, water, food) and those things that promote physical health (e.g. adequate clothing, housing, sanitation). The impact of this sense of environment on health is well documented and has long been a primary focus of nursing care, particularly in public health (Pender & Pender, 1987). A broader view of environment recognizes various psycho-socio-cultural dynamics (Fawcett, 1995). One reviewer of nursing theories suggests "environment" refers to "the recipient's significant others and surroundings, as well as to the setting in which nursing actions occur" (Fawcett, 1989, p. 6). Another reviewer includes "all the internal and external conditions, circumstances, and influences affecting the person" (Wesley, 1992, p. 8).

It is not my intention in this Framework to include every possible use of the term "environment", but rather to describe an environment shared by Christian faith communities. I have identified two major characteristics that describe this shared environment: **Confession** and **Communion**. As we discuss them, I readily acknowledge these characteristics of Christian community are the *ideal*, and may not be evident in *all* church congregations, or in any church at *all* times.

Confession

The image of Catholic churchgoers quietly admitting their wrongdoings to a priest is what comes to mind for many people when they hear the word "**confession**." There are least two different activities defined as confession in The Holy Bible and practiced by people who belong to a faith community: (1). **admission of sin** and (2) **profession of faith** in certain beliefs and doctrines (1 Jn. 1:9; Lockyer, 1986). Theological literature reflects the latter activity in referring to various denominational groups as "confessions" (Lockyer, 1986). Both are relevant to promoting *shalom*-wholeness, individually and corporately, in churches today.

(1) **Admission of sin**. Confession as admission of sin ties in with everything I've said so far about relationships. Right relationships, in both the "vertical" dimension (i.e., with the Triune God) and the "horizontal" dimension (i.e., with self and others), are inherent in this Framework's conceptualization of health as *shalom*-**wholeness** and **stewardship**. Confession as admission of sin means to "agree with" the Triune God about the need for repentance and for restoration of relationship(s) (Lockyer, 1986). Confession is a discipline of disclosing who is really behind one's idealized

images or "masks" (Granberg-Michaelson, 1991). Confession is important in the processes of:

>articulating personal brokenness and pain;
>seeking forgiveness; and
>being restored to harmony with God, self and others.

All of these processes are central to working with people through pastoral care, Christian counseling and spiritual direction. For example, I see them reflected in seven of the twelve "steps" in the "Twelve-Step Programs" for people recovering from (Al-Anon Family Groups, 1990) (See **APPENDIX A**: "The Twelve Steps" and "The Serenity Prayer").

The connection made in The Holy Bible between sin and sickness has already been discussed in the section on Health/*Shalom*-Wholeness. The following quotations draw specific attention to the importance of personal confession of sin to the receiving of forgiveness both from God and from other persons:

>"But if we walk in the light, as He [i.e., God] is in the light, we have fellowship with one another, and the blood of Jesus, His Son, purifies us from all sin. If we claim to be without sin, we deceive ourselves and the truth is not in us. If we confess our sins, He is faithful and just and will forgive us our sins and purify us from all unrighteousness. If we claim we have not sinned, we make Him out to be a liar and His word has no place in our lives" (1 Jn. 1:7-10).

>"Is any one of you sick? He should call the elders of the church to pray over him and anoint him with oil in the name of the Lord. And the prayer offered in faith will make the sick person well; the Lord will raise him up. If he has sinned, he will be forgiven. Therefore confess your sins to each other and pray for each other so that you may be healed. The prayer of a righteous man is powerful and effective" (Jas. 5:14-16).

These passages also emphasize prayer by all persons—for themselves and for one another within the community of faith—to promote healing in every aspect of well-being (spiritual, physical, mental, emotional, social and cultural). All members are to be "pray-ers," especially if they serve in roles such as elder or deacon.

The example and teachings of Jesus closely link the receiving and the giving of forgiveness, such as in Matthew 6:9b-13: "...forgive us our debts, as we also have forgiven our debtors (See **APPENDIX A**: "The Lord's Prayer"). Jesus instructed:

> "When you stand praying, if you hold anything against anyone, forgive him, so that your Father in heaven may forgive you your sins" (Mk. 11:25).
>
> "Do not condemn, and you will not be condemned. Forgive, and you will be forgiven" (Lk. 6:37b).

Forgiveness of one another is also important to promoting healthy relationships within the Body of Christ. Colossians 3:13 is one passage among many which urges Christians to: "Bear with each other and forgive whatever grievances you may have against one another. Forgive as the Lord forgave you."

(2) **Profession of Faith**. Professing belief of certain doctrines or declaring one's faith is the second meaning of confession. In this sense, confession as profession of faith means to affirm or declare one's beliefs openly. The Apostle Paul describes the essential linking of inner belief (in one's "heart") and outer expression (in behavior—with one's mouth):

> "If you confess with your mouth, "Jesus is Lord," and believe in your heart that God raised him from the dead, you will be saved. For it is with your heart that you believe and are justified, and it is with your mouth that you confess and are saved" (Ro. 10:9-10).

It has been stated that "Christian faith is intensely personal, but it is not private" (Moore, 1993, p. 8). Personal beliefs are shared in common with Christians across continents and centuries, including the approximately 1.7 billion other members of the Christian Church worldwide today (Colson, 1992). Great diversity is evident in which aspects of faith are emphasized and in how they are expressed, but agreement on the core set of major beliefs far outweighs doctrinal differences on more minor points (Colson, 1992; Moore, 1993; Pelikan, 1989); (See also **APPENDIX A**: "The Rule of Faith," "The Apostles Creed," and "The Nicene Creed"). Therefore, Christian nurses need to recognize that, despite obvious differences, those who hold a basically Christian worldview have more in common with one another than with those who hold either a predominantly naturalistic, pantheistic or pragmatic secularist worldview (Colson, 1992).

The sharing of faith beliefs in common among Christians contributes to an acknowledgement of shared humanity and likeness in the Church universal and to a sense of belonging within the local church congregation. The public profession of faith (for example, in the universal practices of baptism and communion) brings individual Christians into union with the Triune God, with each other and with the Church of every time and place (World Council of Churches, 1982, p. 3). These practices pay homage to the present Kingdom of God, but they also anticipate the future time when "at the name of Jesus every knee should bow, in heaven and on earth and under the earth, and every tongue confess that Jesus Christ is Lord, to the glory of God the Father" (Php. 2:10-11).

The idea that Christians worldwide are related through their common practices and confessions of faith brings us to the second characteristic that describes their environment: **communion**.

Communion

The term **communion**, like "community," implies relatedness. In this Framework, communion is looked at as three kinds of relationships:

(1) **covenant** relationship with the Triune God,
(2) *koinonia* relationships with other members within The Church, and
(3) **collaborative** relationships within the wider community.

All three are relevant to the promotion of health / *shalom*-wholeness.

(1) **Communion As Covenant Relationship With The Triune God.** Jesus Christ provided a symbolic expression of the personal **"new covenant" relationship** that people could have with God when He shared bread and wine with His disciples. Christians use the term "communion" specifically in referring to the Lord's Supper or Eucharist. (1 Co. 11:25; Heb. 8:6, 13). This public expression of communion as a literal "sharing in common" (Lockyer,

1986) (i.e., of bread and wine) contributes to the sharing of a common faith in Christ in community (1 Co. 10:16-17). This sharing or communion is on both a personal level and a corporate one because the Triune God enters into relationship with people on both levels.

The English word "corporate" derives from the Latin *corpus* meaning "body." The New Testament's reference to the Christian Church as the "Body of Christ" (1 Co. 10:17, 12:27) reflects the corporate nature of the covenant relationship with the Triune God. This relationship between the literal body of Jesus Christ (i.e., resurrected and glorified) (1Ti. 3:16) and the figurative body of His believers (i.e., the Body of Christ, the Church) is viewed as supernatural: a *mystery* beyond human comprehension (Col. 1:18, 1:24b-29; Eph. 5:29-30, 32).

In the Apostles' Creed, the statement "I believe in the holy catholic church, [and] the communion of saints" (The Book of Alternative Services, 1985, p. 189) includes both confession and communion (described as covenant here and as *koinonia* next) (See **APPENDIX A**: "The Apostles' Creed").

(2) **Communion As Koinonia Within The Church Community**. The New Testament Greek word *koinonia*, translated "communion," means "sharing in common" (2 Co. 8:3-5) or "participating in fellowship" (1 Jn. 1:3; Lockyer, 1986). Christians view themselves as members of "God's household" (Eph. 2:19), bonded as a family by their common faith in Christ. The development of such close relationships implies spending significant time together, not only in worship but also in work and play.

In viewing The Church as "Christ's Body," one sees both uniqueness and unity. With Christ as "the head," the mutually-interdependent individual members of the corporate church "body" are to function together as equally necessary and equally valued parts of a unified whole (1 Co. 12:12-27; Eph. 4:3-6; Col. 1:18). These Biblical tenets of equal valuing and vital interdependence within the Christian community are clearly expressed in the following quotation:

> "Those parts of the [human] body that seem to be weaker
> are indispensable, and the parts that we think are less
> honorable we treat with special honor. And the parts

that are unpresentable are treated with special modesty, while our presentable parts need no special treatment. But God has combined the members of the [church] body and has given greater honor to the parts that lacked it, so that there should be no division in the body, but that its parts should have equal concern for each other. If one part suffers, every part suffers with it; if one part is honored, every part rejoices with it. Now you are the body of Christ, and each one of you is a part of it" (1 Co. 12:22-27).

In Judaism, based in the "old covenant," membership in the faith community is exclusive to Abraham's descendants. The "new covenant", on which the Christian Church is founded, is inclusive of whoever believes in Christ (Jn. 3:16). Thus, the early church membership embraced people of diverse nationalities (e.g., Jew, Greek, and Roman) and social groups (e.g., men, women, children, rulers, servants, and slaves) (Gal. 3:26-28). In the terminology of today, this could be deemed a "paradigm shift." An example of this shift, significant particularly from a modern feminist perspective, is the change of the symbol of initiation into the faith community: from circumcision, which is gender-based, to baptism, which is not (Baptist Convention, 1993). Christ came to liberate. Equality is an inherent, core value of the Christian community.

Ideally then, the functions of members within a congregation are gift-based (i.e., personal abilities or spiritual gifts) not power-based, and authority is community-based not individual-based (i.e., authority not over, but on behalf of one another). Within the faith community, individuals' gifts may be discovered, developed, and affirmed in ways that are profoundly empowering (Granberg-Michaelson, 1991). To share one's gifts and resources (e.g., as a parishioner or a Parish Nurse) within the wider community in collaboration with others involved in health promotion in society is also empowering.

(3) **Communion As Collaboration With Others In The Wider Community**. Another aspect of communion is the sharing in Christ's mission and ministry as expressed in humanitarian activities beyond the congregation itself. The presence of Christians, both individually and

corporately, is to be, Biblically speaking, "light" and "salt" (Mt. 5:13-16) which benefit their wider communities in the world. The Christian Church throughout its history has been actively involved in providing many kinds of health-related services. Professionally, Parish Nurses are members of the larger community of all Christian nurses and of the much larger community of all health care workers. The increasing numbers and types of health-promoting programs supported jointly by churches and health care organizations (e.g., hospitals, public health, home care, and continuing care agencies) today reflect the Christian commitment to collaboration with others in society toward a common good.

Inter-relationships of the Framework's Components and Concepts

Much of this Framework can be envisioned as a flower with the **Triune God** as the flower's center, integrating the four petal components made up of the **Person / Parishioner, Health /** *Shalom***-Wholeness, Nurse / Parish Nurse,** and **Community / Parish**. The themes of the **personage** and the **purposes** of the Triune God are evident throughout. The intimate interpersonal relationship of the God-in-three-persons makes relationship itself an integrating concept of all the components. **Co-participation**, viewed as one expression of relationship, is a particularly important concept in the components of **Nurse / Parish Nurse** and **Community / Parish**.

Because **righteousness** and **gracious compassion** characterize the Triune God, the notions of being right with God and of doing right in one's daily life are also imbedded in each component. **Loving** (of the Triune God, oneself, and others) and **caring** (for oneself, others, and the natural world) are key concepts throughout the Framework as well. More specifically, what The Holy Bible refers to as "the fruit of the Holy Spirit"—**love, joy, peace, patience, kindness, goodness, faithfulness, gentleness and self-control** (Gal. 5:22-23a)—is inherent in the larger inter-related concepts of **stewardship** and **ministry**, which are common to all four components.

As the Framework is intended for use within the context of the Christian faith community, it is clearly **centered in Jesus Christ**, including His past, present, and future roles in the Kingdom of God and the Church. An example is the Framework's premise that health/*shalom*-wholeness is experienced in the present life only through personal relationship with Christ.

As another way of describing how inter-related these various concepts are, I wrote a poem (See **APPENDIX B**: "The Faith and Health Framework: A Poem").

CHAPTER 3: NOW WHAT?

CHAPTER 1 answers the *"Why"* and *"How"* questions about the development of the Faith and Health Framework. **CHAPTER 2** describes *"What"* the Framework is. In the final chapter of the book, I invite you to consider the question *"Now what?"* That's the question I asked myself soon after I had completed both the theory *process* and the *product*. My next challenge was to create a three-credit university distance education course in Parish Nursing (Miller, 2000). I had the requisite background as a nurse educator, but I had never before consciously "used" a "nursing theoretical framework." I honestly didn't know when I started how helpful the Faith and Health Framework would be in structuring the course. I began by listing various areas of content and then found they fit logically into modules corresponding to the major components of the Framework. Students' readings, reflections, and other learning activities related aptly too. Clarity in the key concepts and terminology helped integrate the course modules. I sensed a parallel to constructing a building on a solidly laid foundation.

I expect the readers of this book are capable of coming up with innumerable responses to the *"Now what?"* question. To encourage you to "put it on paper," I've left a page blank at the end of this chapter. You may want to pause in your reading and take a few minutes for reflection right now.

As I was writing this chapter, I did some speculating about whom the readers might be and how *they* might "use" the Framework. Recalling the phrase "thinking Christianly about nursing" (JCN, 2002, 19:3), I refocused my speculation to how the *Triune God* might use it *through them*. I have started a list of **examples** you may relate to personally or professionally. I've purposely left spaces for more to be added.

Teachers of Parish Nursing
- Include more in your curriculum re: Christian worldview and theoretical thinking
- Consider revising "accepted" terminology, such as *Parish Nursing* to *ministries of health* (Chase-Ziolek, 2003), to better reflect the underlying thinking re: cultural context of the church.

Students in a Parish Nursing course
- Ask "How would my being a Parish Nurse differ from what I've been doing as a nurse before?"

Instructors of nursing
- Point out in teaching transcultural nursing that the evangelical Christian faith community is a "population" to which "cultural sensitivity" is applicable.
- Openly acknowledge that most patients in hospitals and care facilities are in an older age group which professes faith more than younger age health care workers
- Include more learning activities re: "spiritual care"

Undergraduate nursing students
- Propose alternative topics for course assignments to include a faith and health perspective
- Include spiritual health needs and resources in your assessments of patients.

Graduate nursing students
- In the required nursing theory course identify the underlying worldview of a currently "popular" nursing theory and how it differs from Christian worldview
- Propose a research project that addresses a connection of faith and health
- Critique several Christian nursing conceptual models and do some further development

Parish Nurses
- Use the Framework Figures (e.g. transparencies, posters, etc.) in introductory presentations in churches re: Parish Nursing
- In writing funding proposals cite the Framework and its Biblical references to provide academic credibility and theological grounding

Pastors and Congregational Leaders
- Evaluate the experience of churches with a Parish Nurse on staff re: their mission and ministries of promoting health and healing.

Others Interested in Faith and Health
- Discuss how specific beliefs within your particular faith tradition could either strengthen or weaken someone facing a life-threatening diagnosis or long-term disability.

CONCLUSION

The development of all nursing theory is an open-ended process. It is also a lengthy process. Historically the major conceptual models have taken twenty years to reach the stage they are today. Much collaboration of theorists, educators, researchers and practitioners in diverse settings is required. The field of Parish Nursing is young in years and there is still much to be done in developing its theory base. Publishing this book is my contribution to what is yet to come.

REFERENCES

Adam, E. (1991). To be a nurse (2nd ed.). Philadelphia: W. B. Saunders.

Al-Anon Family Groups. (1990). ...In all our affairs: Making crises work for you. New York: Al-anon Family Group Headquarters.

Anderson, H. (1990). The congregation as a healing resource. In D. S. Browning, T. Jobe, & I. S. Evison (Eds.), Religious and ethical factors in psychiatric practice (pp. 264-286). Chicago: Nelson-Hall & Park Ridge Center for the Study of Health, Faith and Ethics.

Bakken, K. L. (1992). The call to wholeness: Health as a spiritual journey (2nd ed.). New York: Crossroad.

Bakken, K. L., & Hofeller, K. H. (1988). The journey toward wholeness: A Christ-centered approach to health and healing. New York: Crossroad.

Baptist Convention of Ontario and Quebec. (1993). Report of the Working Group on Equality in Ministry (Discussion Paper No. WGEIM Report 1). 217 St. George St., Toronto, ON, M5R 2M2: Author.

Baly, M. (Ed.). (1991). As Miss Nightingale said...Florence Nightingale through her sayings—A Victoria perspective. London: Scutari Press.

Becker, E. (1973). The denial of death. New York: Free Press.

Belleau, M. & Warskow, R. C. (1995). Our journey continues through the art of shared ministry: Rev. Frick and Nurse Frack--Ten years of ministry together. In Proceedings of the Ninth Annual Granger Westberg Parish Nurse Symposium: Parish Nursing--Ministering Through the Arts, (pp. 163-169). Northbrook, IL: National Parish Nurse Resource Center.

Benner, P., & Wrubel, J. (1984). From novice to expert: Excellence and power in clinical nursing practice. Menlo Park, CA: Addison-Wesley.

Bishop, S. (1989). Theory development process. In A. Marriner-Tomey (Ed.), Nursing theorists and their work (pp. 40-61). St. Louis: C. V. Mosby.

Blattner, B. (1981). Holistic nursing. Englewood Cliffs, NJ: Prentice-Hall.

Bloesch, D., Brushaber, G., Bube, R., Holmes, A., Lockerbie, B., Packer, J. I., Ramm, B., & Sire., J. (1982, January). A Christian humanist manifesto. Eternity, pp. 16-22.

The book of alternative services of the Anglican Church of Canada. (1985). Toronto: Anglican Book Centre.

Bouma, H., Diekema, D., Langerak, E., Rottman, T., & Verhey, A. (1989). Christian faith, health and medical practice. Grand Rapids, MI: William B. Eerdmans.

Brittain, J. N. (1986). Theological foundations for spiritual care. Journal of Religion and Health, 25, 107-121.

Brueggemann, W. (1976). Living toward a vision: Biblical reflections on shalom. Philadelphia: United Church Press.

Carson, V. B. (1993). Spirituality: Generic or Christian. Journal of Christian Nursing, 10(1), 24-27.

Christian Medical Commission, World Council of Churches. (1990). Healing and wholeness: The churches' role in health. Geneva, Switzerland: Author.

Christopher, R. (1990). Stewardship and nursing. In R. Stoll (Ed.), Concepts in nursing: A Christian perspective (pp. 123-152). Madison, WI: InterVarsity Christian Fellowship.

Collins, D. R. (1985). Florence Nightingale. Milford, MI: Mott Media.

Colson, C. (1992). The body: Being light in darkness. Dallas: Word.

Coward, H. (1983). Psychology and karma. Philosophy East and West, 33(l), 49-60.

Crabb, L. J. (1987). Understanding people: Deep longings for relationship. Grand Rapids, MI: Zondervan.

Dawn, M. J. (1989). Keeping the Sabbath wholly: Ceasing, resting, embracing, feasting. Grand Rapids, MI: Eerdmans.

Demaray, D. E. (Ed.). (1975). The practice of the presence of God: Brother Lawrence. Grand Rapids, MI: Baker Book House.

Djupe, A. M. (1990). Adjustments, myths and realities of parish nursing. In P. A. Solari-Twadell, A. M. Djupe, & M. A. McDermott (Eds.), Parish nursing: The developing practice (pp. 147-158). Park Ridge, IL: National Parish Nurse Resource Center.

Donley, R., Sr. (1991). Spiritual dimensions of health care. Nursing & Health Care, 12, 178-183.

Droege, T. A. (1995). Congregations as communities of health and healing. Interpretation: A Journal of Bible and Theology, 49, 117-129.

Emblen, J. D. (1992). Religion and spirituality defined according to current use in nursing literature. Journal of Professional Nursing, 8, 41-47.

Evans, A. R., & Small, N. R. (1989). The parish nurse as integrator of health. In Proceedings of the Third Annual Granger Westberg Parish Nurse Symposium: Oneness in Purpose--Diversity in Practice, (pp. 1-30). Northbrook, IL: National Parish Nurse Resource Center.

Fawcett, J. (1989). Analysis and evaluation of conceptual models of nursing (2nd ed.). Philadelphia: F. A. Davis.

Fawcett, J. (1995). Analysis and evaluation of conceptual models in nursing (3rd ed.). Philadelphia: F. A. Davis.

Fordyce, E. M. (1990). Servanthood: Service through nursing. In R. Stoll (Ed.), Concepts in nursing: A Christian perspective (pp. 89-119). Madison, WI: InterVarsity Christian Fellowship.

Gaede, S. D. (1993). When tolerance is no virtue: Political correctness, multiculturism and the future of truth and justice. Downers Grove, IL: InterVarsity Press.

Granberg-Michaelson, K. (1991). Healing community. Geneva, Switzerland: WCC Publications.

Green, J. B. (1994). Caring as gift and goal: Biblical and theological reflections. In S. S. Phillips & P. Benner (Eds.), The crisis of care: Affirming and restoring caring practices in the helping professions (pp. 149-167). Washington, DC: Georgetown University Press.

Guralnik, D. B. (Ed.). (1975). Webster's new world dictionary. Toronto: William Collins & World Publishing.

Gustafson, C. Z. (1993). Parish nursing: A new health partnership in Greater Minnesota. Moorhead, MN: Concordia College.

Harakas, S. S. (1990). Health and medicine in the Eastern Orthodox tradition: Faith, liturgy, and wholeness. New York: Crossroad.

Hauerwas, S. (1990). Naming the silences: God, medicine, and the problem of suffering. Grand Rapids, MI: W. B. Eerdmans.

Haugk, K. C. (1984). Christian caregiving: A way of life. Minneapolis, MN: Augsburg Publishing House.

Health Ministries Association. (1998). Scope and standards of parish nursing practice. Washington DC: American Nurses Publishing.

Henderson, V. (1966). The nature of nursing: A definition and its implications for practice, research, and education. New York: Macmillan.

Holst, L. E. (1982). The hospital chaplain between worlds. In M. E. Marty & K. L. Vaux (Eds.), Health/medicine and the faith traditions: An inquiry into religion and medicine (pp. 293-309). Philadelphia: Fortress Press.

Hustad, D. P. (Ed.). (1992). The worshiping church: A hymnal (4th ed.). Carol Stream, IL: Hope Publishing.

Labonte, R. (1989). Community and professional empowerment. The Canadian Nurse, 85(3), 23-28.

Ladd, G. E. (1974). The presence of the future: The eschatology of biblical realism. Grand Rapids, MI: William B. Eeerdmans.

Lewis, C. S. (1963). The four loves. London: Fontana Books.

Lockyer, H. (Ed.). (1986). Nelson's illustrated Bible dictionary. In PC study Bible for windows 1.4b [Computer program]. Seattle, WA: Biblesoft.

Maton, K. I. (1989). The stress-buffering role of spiritual support: Cross-sectional and prospective investigations. Journal for the Scientific Study of Religion, 28, 310-323.

Maton, K. I., & Rappaport, J. (1984). Empowerment in a religious setting: A multivariate investigation. Prevention in Human Services, 3(2/3), 37-72.

Meleis, A. I. (1991). Theoretical nursing: Development and progress (2nd ed.). Philadelphia: J. B. Lippincott.

Miller, A. B. (1995). Toward a theology of nursing. Journal of Christian Nursing, 12(3), 18-21.

Miller, L.W. (2000) Continuing professional education: A spiritually based program. In Addressing the Spiritual Dimensions of Adult Learning. L.M. English & M. Gillen, (Eds.) San Francisco: Jossey-Bass

Nelson, G. (1990). Pastoral reflections. In P. A. Solari-Twadell, A. M. Djupe, & M. A. McDermott (Eds.), Parish nursing: The developing practice (pp. 277-288). Park Ridge, IL: National Parish Nurse Resource Center.

New international version : The Holy Bible (1984). Colorado Springs: International Bible Society

Numbers, R. L., & Amundsen, D. W. (Ed.). (1986). Caring and curing: Health and medicine in the Western religious traditions. New York: Macmillan.

O'Donnell, J. J. (1989). The mystery of the triune God. New York: Paulist Press.

Ott, P. W. (1991). John Wesley on health as wholeness. Journal of Religion and Health, 30, 43-57.

Pelikan, J. (1989). The Christian tradition: A history of the development of doctrine (Volume V: Christian doctrine and modern culture (since 1700)). Chicago: University of Chicago Press.

Pender, N. J., & Pender, A. R. (1987). Health promotion in nursing practice (2nd ed.). Norwalk, CT: Appleton & Lange.

Peterson, E. H. (1994). Teach us to care and not to care. In S. S. Phillips & P. Benner (Eds.), The crisis of care: Affirming and restoring caring practices in the helping professions (pp. 66-79). Washington, DC: Georgetown University Press.

Robinson, H. W. (1946). Inspiration and revelation in the Old Testament. London: Oxford University Press.

Ryan, J. A. (1990). Society, the parish and the parish nurse. In P. A. Solari-Twadell, A. M. Djupe, & M. A. McDermott (Eds.), Parish nursing: The developing practice (pp. 41-53). Park Ridge, IL: National Parish Nurse Resource Center.

Shelly, J. A. (Ed.). (1993). Teaching spiritual care (2nd ed.). Madison, WI: Nurses Christian Fellowship.

Shelly, J. A. (1994). What is Christian nursing? Journal of Christian Nursing, 11(2), 3-4.

Shelly, J. A. (1995c), Ministry: Vocation of the whole people of God. Unpublished manuscript, The Lutheran Theological Seminary at Philadelphia.

Shelly, J. A., & Miller, A. B. (1991). Values in conflict: Christian nursing in a changing profession. Downers Grove, IL: InterVarsity Press.

Sherburne, B. H. (1990). A biblical view of the person: A basis for value. In R. Stoll (Ed.), Concepts in nursing: A Christian perspective (pp. 15-45). Madison, WI: InterVarsity Christian Fellowship.

Sire, J. W. (1988). The universe next door (2nd ed.). Madison, WI: InterVarsity Press.

Solari-Twadell, P. A., McDermott, M. A., Ryan, J., & Djupe, A. M. (Eds.). (1994). Assuring viability for the future: Guideline development for parish nurse education program. Park Ridge, IL: National Parish Nurse Resource Center.

Solari-Twadell, P. A., & Westberg, G. (1991, September). Body, mind and soul. Health Progress, pp. 24-28.

Stein, J. (Ed.). (1973). Random House dictionary of the English language. New York: Random House.

Stoll, R. I. (1989). Spirituality and chronic illness. In V. B. Carson (Ed.), Spiritual dimensions of nursing practice (pp. 180-214). Toronto: W. B. Saunders.

Striepe, J. M., King, J. M., & Scott, L. (1993). Nurses in the church: Profiles of caring. Journal of Christian Nursing, 10(1), 8-11.

Stumpf, S. E. (1993). Socrates to Sartre: A history of philosophy (5th ed.). Toronto: McGraw-Hill.

Taylor, R. (1986). Christian concepts: Core of professional nursing practice. Andrews University, Berrien Springs, MI: Author.

Thomasma, D. (1994). Beyond the ethics of rightness: The role of compassion in moral responsiblity. In S. S. Phillips & P. Benner (Eds.), The crisis of care: Affirming and restoring caring practices in the helping professions (pp. 123-143). Washington, DC: Georgetown University Press.

Tower, C. (1987, December). Hearts to love, hands to serve: The world of Mother Theresa. Reader's Digest, pp. 170-199.

Travelbee, J. (1966). Interpersonal aspects of nursing (1st ed.). Philadelphia: F. A. Davis.

Tubesing, D. A., & Tubesing, N. L. (1983). The caring question. Minneapolis, MN: Augsburg.

Unger, M. F. (1961). Unger's Bible dictionary (3rd rev. ed.). Chicago: Moody Press.

Watson, J. (1988). <u>Nursing: Human science and human care</u> (2nd ed.). New York: Appleton-Century-Crofts.

Wesley, R. L. (1992). <u>Nursing theories and models</u>. Springhouse, PA: Springhouse.

Westberg, G. (1990). A historical perspective: Wholistic health and the parish nurse. In P. A. Solari-Twadell, A. M. Djupe, & M. A. McDermott (Eds.), <u>Parish nursing: The developing practice</u> (pp. 27-39). Park Ridge, IL: National Parish Nurse Resource Center.

Whitney, D. S. (1991). <u>Spiritual disciplines for the Christian life</u>. Colorado Springs, CO: Navpress.

Wilson, M. (1966). <u>The church is healing</u>. London: SCM Press.

Wolff, H. W. (1974). <u>Anthropology of the Old Testament</u>. Philadelphia: Fortress Press.

World Council of Churches. (1982). <u>Baptism, eucharist and ministry: Faith and order paper no. 111</u>. Toronto: Anglican Book Centre.

Wright, T. (1992). <u>New tasks for a renewed church</u>. London: Hodder and Stoughton.

Wylie, L. J. (1990). The mission of health and the congregation. In P. A. Solari-Twadell, A. M. Djupe, & M. A. McDermott (Eds.), <u>Parish nursing: The developing practice</u> (pp. 11-26). Park Ridge, IL: National Parish Nurse Resource Center.

BIBLIOGRAPHY

OTHER PUBLICATIONS BY THE AUTHOR

Martin, L. B. (1994). Conceptual frameworks for wellness nursing. In Proceedings of the Eighth Annual Westberg Symposium: Ethics and Values--A Framework for Parish Nursing Practice, (pp. 81-94). Northbrook, IL: National Parish Nurse Resource Center.

Martin, L. B. (1996). Parish nursing: Keeping body and soul together. The Canadian Nurse, 92(1), 25-28.

Martin, L. B. (1993). Stress, distress, and eustress. In A. C. Beckingham & B. DuGas (Eds.), Promoting healthy aging: A nursing and community perspective (pp. 303-331). St. Louis: C.V. Mosby.

Miller, L.W. (Winter 1997). Nursing through the lens of faith: A conceptual model. Journal of Christian Nursing. 14 (1), 17-23

Miller, L.W. (1996) A nursing conceptual model grounded in Christian faith. Ph.D. dissertation, University of Victoria, BC.

Miller, L.W. (2000) Continuing professional education: A spiritually based program. In Addressing the Spiritual Dimensions of Adult Learning. L.M. English & M. Gillen, (Eds.) San Francisco: Jossey-Bass

PUBLICATIONS NOT LISTED IN THE REFERENCES

Bergquist, S., & King, J. (1994). Parish nursing: A conceptual framework. Journal of Holistic Nursing, 12, 155-170.

Boland, C. S. (1998). Parish Nursing: Addressing the significance of social support and spirituality for sustained health-promoting behaviors in the elderly. Journal of Holistic Nursing, 16(3), 355-369.

Carson, V. B. (Ed.). (1989c). Spiritual dimensions of nursing practice. Philadelphia: W. B. Saunders.

Carson, V. & Koenig, H. (2002) Parish Nursing: Stories of service and care. Philadelphia: Templeton Foundation Press.

Chase-Ziolek, M. (1999). The meaning and experience of health ministry within the culture of a congregation with a parish nurse. Journal of Transcultural Nursing, 10(1), 46-55.

Chase-Ziolek, M. (2003). Rethinking our terms: Health Ministry or Ministry of Health? Journal of Christian Nursing,20(2),21-22.

Evans, A. R. (1995). The church as an institution of health. Interpretation: A Journal of Bible and theology, 49(2)(April), 158-171.

Fitchett, G. (1993). Assessing spiritual needs: A guide for caregivers. Minneapolis, MN: Augsburg.

Gibble, J. A. (1993). The lafiya guide: A congregational handbook for whole-person health ministry. Elgin, IL: Association of Brethren Caregivers.

Holifield, E.B. (1996). Health and medicine in the Methodist tradition. New York: Crossroad.

Johnson, D. E. (1992). Development of theory: A requisite for nursing as a primary health profession. In L. H. Nicoll (Ed.), Perspectives on nursing theory (pp. 335-347). Philadelphia: J. B. Lippincott.

Karns, P. S. (1991). Building a foundation for spiritual care. Journal of Christian Nursing 8(3), 10-13.

Kelsey, M. (1995). Healing and Christianity. Minneapolis: Augsburg.

Koenig, H., M. McCullough and D. Larson. (2001) Handbook of religion and health. Oxford University Press.

Marty, M., & Vaux, K. (1982). Health/Medicine and the faith traditions: An inquiry into religion and medicine.

Miller, B. J. (2002). Who needs theories, anyhow?. Journal of Christian Nursing. 19 (3), 6-10.

Miskelly, S. (1995). A parish nursing model: Applying the community health nursing process in a church community. Journal of Community Health Nursing, 12(1), 1-14.

Myers, M.E. (2002). The integrative parish nursing model: A theoretical framework for practice, education & research. Toronto: Opus Wholistic Publications.

Myers, M.E. (2002). Parish nursing speaks: The voices of those who practice, facilitate, and support parish nursing. Toronto: Opus Wholistic Publications.

Nicoll, L. H. (Ed.). (1992). Perspectives on nursing theory (2nd ed.). Philadelphia: J. B. Lippincott

Nurses Christian Fellowship, Ad Hoc Committee. (1985). This we believe: A Christian philosophy of nursing. Madison, WI: Author.

O'Brien, M. E. (1999). Spirituality in nursing: Standing on holy ground. Sudbury, MA: Jones & Bartlett Publishers.

O'Brien, M.E. (2003). Parish nursing: Healthcare ministry within the church. Sudbury, MA: Jones & Bartlett Publishers.

Patterson, D. (2003). The essential parish nurse: ABCs for congregational health ministry. Pilgrim Press.

Rethemeyer, A. & Wehling, B. (2004). How are we doing? Measuring the effectiveness of parish nursing. Journal of Christian Nursing. 21(2), 10-12.

Roach, S. (1992). The human act of caring. Ottawa: Canadian Hospital Association.

Rydholm, L. (1997). Patient-focused care in parish nursing. Holistic Nursing Practice, 11(3), 47-60.

Schuler, L. (2000). Parish nursing is ministry. Journal of Christian Nursing, 17(1), 23.

Schwank, M.J., Weis, D., & Matheus, R. (1996). Parish nursing: ministry of health. Geriatric Nursing, 17, 11-13

Sellers, S. C., & Haag, B. (1998). Spiritual nursing interventions. Journal of Holistic Nursing, 16(3), 338-354.

Sensenig, J. E. (1993). Nurse in the congregation: A guidebook for planning health ministries in mennonite churches. New Holland, PA: Mennonite Mutual Aid.

Shelly, J. A. (1999). <u>Called to care: A Christian theology of nursing</u>. Downers Grove, IL: InterVarsity Press.

Shelly, J.A. (ed) (2002). <u>Nursing in the church.</u> Madison, WI: NCF Press

Shelly, J. A. (2000). <u>Spiritual care: A guide to caregivers</u>. Downers Grove, IL: InterVarsity Press.

Smith, S. D. (2000). Parish nursing: A call to integrity. <u>Journal of Christian Nursing, 17</u>(1 (Winter)), 18-20.

Smith, S. D. (ed) (2003) <u>Parish nursing: A handbook for the new millennium</u>. Binghamton, NY: The Haworth Pastoral Press.

Smucker, C. J. (1989). Church nurse: Caring for a congregation. <u>Journal of Christian Nursing</u>, 6(1), 32-33.

Solari-Twadell, P. A., & McDermott, M. A. (Eds.). (1999). <u>Parish nursing: Promoting whole person health within faith communities</u>. Thousand Oaks, CA: Sage Publications.

Stegmeir, D. (2002). Faith & nursing: Adjusting nursing theories to Christian beliefs. <u>Journal of Christian Nursing</u>. 19 (3), 11-15.

Stoll, R. I. (1979). Guidelines for spiritual assessment. <u>American Journal of Nursing, 79</u>, 1574-1577.

Stoll, R. I. (Ed.). (1990). <u>Concepts in nursing: A Christian perspective</u>. Madison, WI: InterVarsity Christian Fellowship.

Tuck, I. & Wallace, D. (2000). Exploring parish nursing from an ethnographic perspective. <u>Journal of Christian Nursing</u>, 11 (4), 280-289.

United Methodist Church. (1995). <u>Congregational health ministries resource packet</u>. New York: Author

Vandecreek, L. et al (eds.) (2002). <u>Parish nurses, health care chaplains and community clergy: Navigating the maze of professional relationship</u>. Binghamton, NY: The Haworth Pastoral Press.

Warren, R. (2002). <u>The purpose driven life: What on earth am I here for?</u>. Grand Rapids, MI: Zondervan.

Westberg, G. (1986). The role of congregations in preventive medicine. Journal of Religion and Health, 25(3), 1-4.

Westberg, G. E., & McNamara, J. W. (1990). The parish nurse: Providing a minister of health for your congregation. Minneapolis: Augsburg Fortress.

Faith and Health: A Framework for Christian Nurses

APPENDIX A: TEXTUAL MATERIALS

Historical Background of Parish Nursing

Promoting health and healing in the Christian faith community through designated members, particularly deacons, began in Apostolic times and is evident in the New Testament record and throughout church history (Numbers & Amundsen, 1986). The modern profession of nursing itself traces its own history from early Church roots and on through the nursing work in later centuries of Catholic nuns, Lutheran deaconesses, and Florence Nightingale.

Parish Nursing emerged from a project of church-based "wholistic health centers" (Westberg, 1990, p. 27) envisioned in the late 1960's by the Reverend Granger Westberg, a clergyman with a joint appointment as Hospital Chaplain and Professor in the University of Chicago Medical School. These centers employed teams consisting of a family physician, a pastor, and a nurse in a whole-person health care approach. Dozens of these centers were set up over the next fifteen years, including at least one in Canada (at the First Lutheran Church, Vancouver, BC), but most were not economically viable (Martin, 1996). Evaluators of the centers observed that the nurses served as "translators" (Westberg, 1990, p. 28) because of their understanding of both the humanities and the sciences, and of the languages of both religion and medicine.

In 1984, Westberg observed a wellness clinic project in Tucson in which a nurse educator from the University of Arizona served alone as a Minister of Health in a local Lutheran church. She provided health promotion seminars and personal health counseling, which included physical examinations. "Tremendously impressed with the success of the Tucson venture," (Westberg & McNamara, 1987, p. 29) implemented the first parish nurse project in 1985 by placing six nurses in Chicago-area churches in conjunction with the Lutheran General Hospital, in Park Ridge, IL.

Through the parish nurse project, as in the wholistic health center project that preceded it, Westberg hoped to "stimulate the dialogue between science and religion at the grass-roots level" (Westberg & McNamara, 1987, p. 6). Viewing health as "a natural part of the vocabulary of the Bible and of Christian theology," he proposed that parish nurses could "assist in encouraging people toward the whole-person goals of the highest scriptural injunctions" (Westberg, 1990, p. 37). He saw the role as "basically reaching out for more whole-person ways of ministering to people who are hurting" (Westberg, 1990, p. 38). He had also observed, particularly in the process of interviewing applicants for the initial parish nurse positions, that most of the candidates indicated that their decision to enter nursing was strongly motivated by "a desire to incorporate the spiritual dimension into their work" (Westberg, 1990, p. 31). He noted that they were "interested in a type of nursing which would allow the kind of creativity they had always longed for" and he found them "stimulated by the potential of a whole-person approach" (Westberg, 1990, p. 30).

Westberg (1990) argued there was a direct relationship between personal health/illness and personal outlook/philosophy of life, and hence argued that "religious institutions must be integrated into the health care system" (p. 33). He saw churches as the "natural setting" (p. 37)—and "spiritually mature" parish nurses as the "natural organizers" (p. 33)—for promoting the integration and well-being of body, mind, and spirit. Thus, the pivotal role of the parish nurse became that of an "integrator of faith and health" (p. 37).

Interest in the Lutheran General project grew so rapidly that the National Parish Nurse Resource Center was established IN 1986 to handle the flood of enquiries for information and consultation. In 1996, its name was changed to The International Parish Nurse Resource Center (IPNRC), and in 2002 the IPNRC was reorganized and relocated to St. Louis, Missouri (see **APPENDIX D: RESOURCES**). Also expanding is the Health Ministries Association (HMA), a closely affiliated non-profit, ecumenical, inter-faith and inter-disciplinary membership organization formed in 1989 (See **APPENDIX D: RESOURCES**). One task of this organization that is relevant to Parish Nursing is the setting of "Standards of Practice" as a nursing specialty recognized by the American Nurses Association (Health Ministries Association, 1998).

In 1992, the Carter Center at Emory University, Atlanta, established the Interfaith Health Program to encourage faith groups to "improve the individual and collective health of the local and global communities they serve" (Droege, 1995, pp. 122-123). (See **APPENDIX D: RESOURCES**).

No nursing practice equivalent to Parish Nursing in the U.S.A. had been reported in Canada prior to my article in the January 1996 issue of The Canadian Nurse (Martin, 1996).   That report identified three Canadian nurses who had completed Parish Nursing educational programs in the U.S.A., only one of whom then held a designated parish nurse position. In 1995 a pilot project was begun in Ontario, and by 1998 there were educational programs being offered through the University of Alberta and St. Francis Xavier University, Nova Scotia. Also in 1998 a Canadian Parish Nursing Ministry Steering Committee and Forum founded what is now a national organization—The Canadian Association for Parish Nursing Ministry) (See **APPENDIX D: RESOURCES**).

From its inception, Parish Nursing has been described as a "ministry" of health promotion, not as a "hands-on" health care service (Solari-Twadell & Westberg, 1991, p. 25). The role is a developing one; in that each parish nurse's specific roles are determined by the composition and concerns of the local church congregation and the community it serves (Solari-Twadell, Djupe, & McDermott, 1990). The role generally includes, however, a range of functions such as health educator, personal health counselor, health advocate, trainer/coordinator of volunteers, facilitator/coordinator of support groups, and referral agent/liaison with community resources (Striepe, King, & Scott, 1993; Health Ministries Association, 1998). Some churches have developed "ministers of health" (Solari-Twadell, 1990, p. 58) (not necessarily nurses) or a "wellness committee" (Solari-Twadell & Westberg, 1991, p. 25) within a concept of congregational wholistic health and healing ministries (Droege, 1995).   The Parish Nurse has often been described as an "integrator of faith and health" (Health Ministries Association, 1998). The foundational context for the role, however, is that of the church as a "health and healing place" (Wylie, 1990, p. 11).

The Apostles' Creed

from (The Book of Alternative Services, 1985, p. 189)

I believe in God, the Father almighty, creator of heaven and earth.
I believe in Jesus Christ, his only Son, our Lord.
He was conceived by the power of the Holy Spirit and born of the Virgin Mary. He suffered under Pontius Pilate, was crucified, died, and was buried.
He descended to the dead.
On the third day he rose again. He ascended into heaven, and is seated at the right hand of the Father.
He will come again to judge the living and the dead.
I believe in the Holy Spirit, the holy catholic Church, the communion of saints, the forgiveness of sins, the resurrection of the body, and the life everlasting. Amen.

The Nicene Creed

from (The Book of Alternative Services, 1985, p. 188)

We believe in one God, the Father, the Almighty, maker of heaven and earth, of all that is, seen and unseen.
We believe in one Lord, Jesus Christ, the only Son of God, eternally begotten of the Father, God from God, Light from Light, true God from true God, begotten, not made, of one being with the Father.
Through him all things were made.
For us and for our salvation he came down from heaven: by the power of the Holy Spirit he became incarnate from the Virgin Mary, and was made man.
For our sake he was crucified under Pontius Pilate; he suffered death and was buried.
On the third day he rose again in accordance with the scriptures; he ascended into heaven and is seated at the right hand of the Father.
He will come again in glory to judge the living and the dead, and his kingdom will have no end.

We believe in the Holy Spirit, the Lord, the giver of life, who proceeds from
the Father.
With the Father and the Son he is worshipped and glorified.
He has spoken through the prophets.
We believe in one holy catholic and apostolic Church.
We acknowledge one baptism for the forgiveness of sins.
We look for the resurrection of the dead, and the life of the world to come.
Amen.

The Lord's Prayer

(from Mt.hew 6:9b-13)   Our Father in heaven, hallowed be your name, your
kingdom come, your will be done on earth as it is in heaven. Give us today
our daily bread. Forgive us our debts, as we also have forgiven our debtors.
And lead us not into temptation, but deliver us from the evil one. [*some late
manuscripts include*: for yours is the kingdom and the power and the glory
forever. Amen.]

The Prayer of the Trinity
from (Wright, 1992, p. 180).

Father almighty, maker of heaven and earth: Set up your kingdom in our
midst.
Lord Jesus Christ, Son of the living God: Have mercy on me, a sinner.
Holy Spirit, breath of the living God: Renew me and all the world.

The Westminister Confession II,1
from (Sire, 1988, p. 222)

There is but one living and true God, who is infinite in being and perfection,
a most pure spirit, invisible, without body, parts or passions, immutable,
immense, eternal, incomprehensible, almighty; most wise, most holy, most

free, most absolute, working all things according to the counsel of his own immutable and most righteous will, for his own glory; most loving, gracious, merciful, long-suffering, abundant in goodness and truth, forgiving iniguity, transgression and sin; the rewarder of them that diligently seek him; and withal most just and terrible in his judgements; hating all sin, and who will by no means clear the guilty."

The Rule of Faith
from (Colson, 1992, p. 108)

*God the creator exists in three persons, Father, Son, and Holy Spirit.
*Born of the virgin, He suffered, died, rose again, and was exalted at the right hand of the Father from whence He will come again.
*The Holy Spirit brings the benefits of Christ's saving work to people who believe in Him
*Christians are expected to unite with a local church, submit to the authority of bishops and elders, live a holy life conducive to the spread of the gospel.
*God will judge the world and receive His own at the end of history.

Florence Nightingale Pledge
from (a bookmark, 1963, Philadelphia, Quality Weaving Co)

I solemnly pledge myself before God and in the presence of this assembly: To pass my life in purity and to practice my profession faithfully.
I will abstain from whatever is deleterious and mischievous,
and will not take or knowingly administer any harmful drug.
I will do all in my power to maintain and elevate the standard of my profession, and will hold in confidence all personal matters committed to my keeping and all family affairs coming to my knowledge in the practice of my profession. With loyalty will I endeavor to aid the physician in his work and devote myself to the welfare of those committed to my care.

A Quotation of Florence Nightingale

cited in (Baly, 1991, p. 68).

"Nursing is an art, and if it is to be made an art, it requires as exclusive a devotion, as hard a preparation, as any painter's or sculptor's work. For what is having to do with dead canvas or cold marble compared with having to do with the living body, the temple of God's spirit

The Twelve Steps

from (Al-Anon Groups, 1990, p. 239)

1. We admitted we were powerless over alcohol-that our lives had become unmanageable.
2. Came to believe that a Power greater than ourselves could restore us to sanity.
3. Made a decision to turn our will and our lives over to the care of God as we understood Him.
4. Made a searching and fearless moral inventory of ourselves.
5. Admitted to God, to ourselves, and to another human being the exact nature of our wrongs.
6. Were entirely ready to have God remove all these defects of character.
7. Humbly asked Him to remove our shortcomings.
8. Made a list of all person we had harmed, and became willing to make amends to them all.
9. Made direct amends to such people whereve possible, except when to do so would injure them or others.
10. Continued to take personal inventory and when we were wrogn promptly admitted it.
11. Sought through prayer and meditation to improve our conscious contact with God as we understood Him, praying only for knowledge of His will for us and the power to carry that out.
12. Have had a spiritual awakening as the result of these Steps, we tried to carry this message to others, and to practice these principles in all our affairs.

The Serenity Prayer
By Reinhold Neibuhr (public domain)

God, grant me the serenity to accept the things I cannot change,
The courage to change the things I can,
And the wisdom to know the difference
Living one day at a time, enjoying one moment at a time,
Accepting hardship as a pathway to peace,
Taking this sinful world as it is, not as I would have it.
Trusting that you will make all things right if I surrender to your will,
So that I may be reasonably happy in this life and supremely happy with you
forever in the next.   Amen

Hymn of St. Patrick
from (Wright, 1992, pp. 175,176).

I bind unto myself this day the strong name of the Trinity;
By invocation of the same, the three in one and one in three.
Of whom all nature hath creation, eternal Father, Spirit, Word.
Praise to the Lord of my salvation; salvation is of Christ the Lord.

I bind this day to me for ever, by power of faith, Christ's incarnation,
His baptism in Jordan river, his death on cross for my salvation;
His bursting from the spiced tomb, his riding up the heavenly way,
His coming at the day of doom, I bind unto myself today.

I bind unto myself today the virtues of the star-lit heaven,
The glorious sun's life-giving ray, the whiteness of the moon at even,
The flashing of the lightning free, the whirling wind's tempestuous shocks,
The stable earth, the deep salt sea around the old eternal rocks.

I bind unto myself today the power of God to hold and lead,
His eye to watch, his might to stay, his ear to hearken to my need,
The wisdom of my God to teach, his hand to guide, his shield to ward,
The word of God to give me speech, his heavenly host to be my guard.

Christ be with me, Christ within me, Christ behind me, Christ before me,
Christ beside me, Christ to win me, Christ to comfort and restore.
Christ beneath me, Christ above me, Christ in quiet, Christ in danger,
Christ in hearts of all that love me, Christ in mouth of friend and stranger.

I bind unto myself this day the strong name of the Trinity;
By invocation of the same, the three in one and one in three.
Of whom all nature hath creation, eternal Father, Spirit, Word.
Praise to the Lord of my salvation; salvation is of Christ the Lord.

The Servant Song

by Richard Gillard
from (Granberg-Michaelson, 1991, p. 37)

Beloved let me be your servant,
let me be as Christ to you;
pray that I may have the grace
to let you be my servant, too.

We are pilgrims on a journey,
we are family on the road;
we are here to help each other
walk the mile and bear the load.

I will hold the Christ-light for you
in the night time of your fear;
I will hold my hand out to you,
speak the peace you long to hear.

I will weep when you are weeping;
when you laugh I'll laugh with you.
I will share your joy and sorrow
'til we've seen this journey through.

Faith and Health: A Framework for Christian Nurses

APPENDIX B

The Faith And Health Framework: A POEM ©
by Lynda W. Miller

-The Triune God-
Infinite. Intimate.
creating, sustaining, restoring, enjoying.
Love-in-Three Persons
always there.

-Human Being-
dependent, dignified.
living, needing, struggling, changing.
Body-Soul-Spirit
Shalom-wholeness.

-Community of Faith-
believing, bonded.
worshipping, learning, serving, healing.
Light and Salt
'til Christ returns.

-Parish Nurse-
called, competent.
listening, helping, encouraging, connecting
Faith and Health.
Compassionate care.

APPENDIX C: LISTS OF REVIEWERS AND PRAYER PARTNERS

REVIEWERS OF THE 1ST DRAFT OF THE FRAMEWORK

Judith Anderson (School of Nursing, Clackamas College; Northwest Parish Nurse Ministries, Portland, OR)

Dr. Kenneth Bakken (Director, St.Luke Health Ministries, Bellevue, WA)

Dr. Verna Carson (Tender Loving Care-Staff Builders Home Care, Baltimore, MD)

Dr. Thomas Droege (Inter-Faith Health Program, The Carter Center, Emory University, Atlanta, GA)

Dr. Josephine Flaherty (Former Principal Nursing Officer, Health Canada, Ottawa, ON)

Dr. Edwin Hui (Faculty, Regent College, Vancouver, BC)

Helene Kahlsdorf (College of Nursing, University of North Dakota; Olive Tree Wellness Ministries, LaPorte, MN)

Dr. Phyllis Karns (Dean, School of Nursing, Baylor University, Baylor,TX)

Marabel Kersey (Coordinator, Community Parish Nurse Program, Methodist Health Network, Des Moines, Iowa)

Rev. Alistair Petrie (former Rector, Brentwood Anglican Chapel, Brentwood Bay, BC)

Dr. Judy Shelly (Publications Director, Nurses Christian Fellowship, Madison, WI)

Dr. James Sire (Senior Editor, Inter-Varsity Press, Downers Grove, IL)

Dr. Norma Small (Former Dean, Graduate Program, Georgetown University School of Nursing, Baltimore, MD; Director, Concerned Care Management & Consultation, Johnstown, PA)

Annette Stixrud (Coordinator, Northwest Parish Nurse Ministries, Portland OR)

Dr. Ruth I. Stoll (School of Nursing, Messiah College, Grantham, PA)

Dr. Rilla Taylor (Chair, Nursing Dept., Andrews University, Berrien Springs, MI)

Rev. Granger Westberg (Founder, National Parish Nurse Resource Center, Park Ridge, IL)

MY "PRAYER PARTNERS"

Carol Bailey, RN, MSN
Michael Beebe, RN, Ph.D.
Rob Calnan, RN, Ph.D.
Mary Dixon, retired nurse-midwife
Carrol Duke, RN
Kay Eggert
Lorene Freeman, RN, MSN
Lucille Gracey
Jeanette Harrison
Grace Hodgins, RN
Harry Life
Mae Meller, RN, BSN
Jan Morton
Betty Anne Smith, RN, BSN
Marian Templeton, RN
Patricia O'Meara Thompson, RN.

APPENDIX D: RESOURCES

ORGANIZATIONS:

1. **The Canadian Association for Parish Nursing Ministry** (a membership organization); annual education conference; 56 Thames St., Ingersoll, ON N5C 2S9 519-485-3390 parishnursing@capnm.ca   www.capnm.ca

2. **Health Ministries Association**, (a membership organization) developed Scope and Standards of Practice; annual national conference; 295 W. Crossville Rd., Suite 130, Roswell, GA 30075   1-800-280-9919 www.hmassoc.org

3. **International Parish Nurse Resource Center**, Deaconess Parish Nurse Ministries, 475 E. Lockwood Avenue, St. Louis, MO 63119; sponsors the annual Westberg Symposium. 314-918-2559 www.parishnurses.org arethemeyer@eden.edu

4. **Australian Faith Community Nurses Association (AFCNA)**, contact Anne VanLoon, South Australia, P.O. Box 2707, Kent Town, South Australia 5071. Phone (08) 8278 8274. www.afcna.org.au VanLoon.Anne@rdns.sa.gov.au

5. **Nurses Christian Fellowship USA,** PO Box 7895, Madison, WI 53707-7895. 608-274-4823 Ext. 402 www.ncf.org ncf@ivcf.org

6. **Nurses Christian Fellowship Canada,** Anne Hawes, Director; IVCF Canada, 64 Prince Andrew Place, Toronto, M3C 2H4. 1-800-668-9766. www.ivcf.ca (Adult/Vocation ministry). ncf@ivcf.ca

7. **The Interfaith Health Program**, Rollins School of Public Health of Emory University, Decatur, GA; contact Gary Gunderson 404-592-1465 www.ihpnet.org

FAITH & HEALTH FRAMEWORK RESOURCES

Stained Glass Figures designed for use as posters, overhead transparencies or other formats may be obtained through Dr. Lynda Miller. 250-652-0658 lwmiller@telus.net

Lapel pins in a design based on **Figure 5** are available to any one who has completed a parish nursing educational program that includes the Faith & Health Framework. Contact Dr. Lynda Miller directly for description and current pricing. 250-652-0658 lwmiller@telus.net

JOURNAL:

The Journal of Christian Nursing , JCN, NCF Press, P.O. Box 7895, Madison, WI 5370 –7895, 608-274-4823, Ext. 401; **jcn@ivcf.org   www.ncf-jcn.org**

VIDEOS:

"The Healing Team: An introduction to health ministry and parish nursing" available from The International Parish Nurse Resource Center, Deaconess Parish Nurse Ministries, 475 E. Lockwood Avenue, St. Louis, MO 63119 www.ipnrc.parishnurses.org 314-918-2559

"Parish Nurses On Call for Tomorrow" (2000) 9 minutes; $15 plus postage; Oshawa, Ontario: InterChurch Health Ministries 905-436-1572 info@ichm.on.ca

GUIDES FOR PRACTICE AND EDUCATION:

The Canadian Association for Parish Nursing Ministry (2004). Guide for Parish Nursing Core Competencies for Basic Parish Nurse Educational Program. and Standards of Practice for Parish Nursing Ministry (2004).;

contact CAPN: 56 Thames St. S., Ingersoll, ON N5C 2S9   519-485-3390
parishnursing@capnm.ca   www.capnm.ca

Health Ministries Association. A Guide to Developing a Health Ministry.
Manual. Roswell, GA   1-800-280-9919 www.hmaassoc.org

Health Ministries Association. (1998) Scope and Standards of Parish Nursing
Practice. Washington DC: American Nurses Publishing. www.hmaassoc.org

InterChurch Health Ministries Handbook and Resources Manual. Oshawa,
ON Canada: ICHM 905-436-1572   info@ichm.on.ca

COMPUTER PROGRAM:

Biblesoft.   PC Study Bible [Computer program]. Seattle, WA: Biblesoft:
22014 7th Ave. S., 98198.

ISBN 1412009768